THE NATURAL FOOD REDUCING DIET

by Harry Preston
In collaboration with
Emil J. Halley, M.D.

CASTLE BOOKS / NEW JERSEY

CONTENTS

Introduction

Emil J. Halley, M.D.

Over the years, many patients have come to me with a weight problem. There have been those who wanted to gain, but the majority, like so many Americans, have suffered from overweight; with few exceptions, they have usually expected some sort of medical miracle that would restore them to a normal weight balance practically overnight. Like too many unsuspecting consumers, they have been misled by exaggerated advertising claims for reducing aids, and overlook a basic proven fact: that weight gains and losses are governed primarily by the quantity and quality of food we consume.

Obviously, nobody puts on twenty pounds in one week; similarly, no one can hope to take off that much weight in a few days. The body must be given a chance to get back to normal in a manner that is natural and which will usually result in a proper weight balance being maintained after the undesired pounds are removed.

I have often heard people complain they went on a diet and lost weight, but a month later, it was back again. Very often, such "diets" turn out to be little more than enforced starvation resulting from taking an appetite depressant together with large amounts of water or fruit juices. The pounds melt away, but when the person goes back to his former food intake, the body responds and the weight naturally returns.

Thousands of Americans go through this "off-again, on-again" type of weight variation when they could more easily maintain their desired normal proportions through paying proper attention to what they eat; for in truth, our bodies reflect our eating habits.

Anyone who shovels too much of the wrong food into his stomach is going to find a spare tire inflating his waist, together with the many unpleasant results of an improper diet.

Many patients have told me they consider themselves quite healthy, even though they are overweight, another indication of how few people associate weight with health. I have always maintained that improper weight is an unhealthy condition, and health is achieved more easily (and cheaply!) by eating the right foods than by dashing to the drugstore or the doctor for medications to hopefully correct the results of our indiscretions at the dinner table.

Many of us have developed bad eating habits, mostly through temptation. Today's array of foods is the greatest in history, and certainly the most appealing. Fluffy meringue six inches high on a chiffon chocolate pie is hard to turn down; it looks good and tastes delicious. Yet one fresh apple or a quartered orange holds more nourishment and food value, and contains not one of the dozen or so chemical emulsifiers that are responsible for the texture and size of the artificially-flavored mixture in the pie shell! The apple or orange will sit well on the stomach; the pie can easily have one reaching for the Alka-Seltzer an hour afterwards, thereby compounding the ultimate harm to the digestion.

Eating is a natural instinct; without it, we would waste away and die. But today's eating habits are not always governed by our need for sustenance, but more often for self-gratification. Exotic concoctions like the pie described above possess a definite sensual appeal. Psychologists have proven that too often our desire for certain foods, together with our between-meal snacks, is sparked by emotional tensions rather than the need for food.

Men and women who experience frustration in their sex lives, for example, often turn to eating as a substitute satisfaction. There is a saying that an active sex life results in a trim body; the explanation is rooted less in the exercise factor than in psychology: When our desires are satisfied in the bedroom, we do not seek consolation in the kitchen!

I mention this fact because, apart from the physical aspects of weight control, the psychological factors are also very important. The dictionary defines health as "soundness of body or mind"; I prefer "body *and* mind", because the two are so closely interrelated that they cannot work independently. Physical and mental health go hand in hand, especially in the attainment of ideal body weight.

Our mental attitudes have a profound effect upon the reaction of the body to the food we eat, and upon the body chemistry. An unhealthy state of mind, such as anger and fear, causes the body to produce secretions which affect the digestion of food, as well as the metabolic processes. A housewife who has had a violent argument and stormed into the kitchen to gorge herself on cookies and ice cream can easily end up with a few extra pounds as well as a bad case of indigestion. Continued aggravation can ultimately result in stomach ulcers and hypertension. You might claim it is only natural to become emotional at times, which is true; but to take out our frustrations in food is only asking for trouble, both from a digestive as well as a weight standpoint.

You will note that I am using the word "natural" quite often, and for a purpose. Just as our *natural*, calm emotional state aids our absorption of food, so also does our physical state benefit from the intake of *natural* food in contrast to the preponderance of processed foods presently available and generally used.

Unfortunately, the bulk of food products today contains little of the basic natural ingredients we need, and an alarming amount of chemicals, preservatives and emulsifiers which the food industry considers essential for economic reasons; that is, without these artificial additives, certain processed foods would not look as appealing (and therefore would not sell as well) nor would they last very long on the grocer's shelf.

The food industry is to be complimented for

the virtually infinite variety of items to tempt the palate. But while most of these tickle the taste buds, they do not always provide the basic nourishment essential to good health, and in this area, the food manufacturers have often come under the suspicious scrutiny of the Food and Drug Administration. The artificial sweetener, cyclamate, is a good example of a food additive that was proven to be hazardous to health; how many more chemicals currently in use may soon suffer a similar fate?

As a physician, I am especially aware of the progress of science and the wonders of modern technology, but in the matter of food, I adhere to the premise that what nature has provided for our sustenance has yet to be improved upon as a source of growth, energy and daily maintenance of the human body.

Bread is a prime example of how the food industry has taken a basic food staple and changed it into a product which can be sorely lacking in natural nutritive value. I am not referring now to the multitudinous display of breads, but to the basic product itself, which has been possibly the most commonly eaten food throughout history.

What *is* bread? Originally, when the wheat matured naturally in the field, the harvest was taken to a mill where the grains were crushed between millstones to produce flour. During storage, the flour would whiten naturally with age, after which it was combined with yeast, eggs and milk to produce bread that was rich in minerals and natural vitamins, especially the B complex. A slice of such bread would constitute a valuable supplement to any meal. Unfortunately, bread such as I have just described is difficult to find today.

The modern milling process breaks the wheat into its three component parts: the husk, the endosperm and the germ. The husk, or outer part, contains natural vitamins and minerals; the germ contains protein and minerals; the endosperm is the least nutritious part, yet this is the substance from which is made the low-grade, non-nutritious white flour used for most bread and baked goods produced today in mass quantities. To compensate for all the goodness that is inevitably removed in the refining processes, the flour is treated with "improvers" such as persulphate, bromate, iodate and nitrogen trichloride to make it more glutenous. Bleachers and softening agents are also added, together with emulsifiers to make the bread stay soft, even when it may get moldy. The modern bread-making process uses more than 90 ingredients that do not have to be identified on the label.

Advertisements for a certain brand of bread stress the beneficial substances added to the product. However, in the refining process, more than 22 natural nutrients are removed, and no amount of artificial enrichers are able to equal the nutritive value of the real thing.

The industrial chemists are to be congratulated for helping produce a substance more economically appealing to the bakeries, who are able to market a large loaf for around 35 cents. Cheap, yes. Nutritious? Not very. Oddly enough, I have had patients who drive the most expensive cars available balk at the idea of spending 55 cents for high-quality bread that contains a far more respectable proportion of natural goodness than the cheaper mass-produced varieties. "Bread is bread," some people claim, but this is not so. As with most of our processed foods today, many natural food elements are missing in the majority of breads produced in mass quantities.

Which is why I recommend natural foods, not only for top nutrition, but to help those with a weight problem get their body metabolism back to normal.

The real secret to maintaining proper weight lies in the biochemical uniqueness of each individual, which means everyone has his or her particular way of reacting to food consumed. On identical diets, two people may display a wide variance in weight loss due to individual responses to nourishment.

While many factors are involved, much of this variance can be traced to bodily reactions to the additives and preservatives found in most processed foods, together with the lack of balance of natural nutrients. While one cannot possibly prescribe a diet without a personal examination of the individual, there are aspects of controlling weight that are affected by the intake of a *naturally* balanced combination of essential foods. Briefly, with the right amounts of all the needed natural foods, the body metabolism will ultimately adjust and a normal weight balance will result, provided sensible amounts of food are consumed and no abnormal gland functioning or other pathological symptoms are present.

In other words, if you are a normally healthy person, the right amounts of the right foods will enable you to maintain proper body weight. Just as in a later chapter we detail the importance of limiting calories and carbohydrates in losing weight, this factor is significant in *maintaining* your desired weight level after the excess pounds have disappeared.

When insufficient natural nutrients and too many artificial chemical compounds are present in a diet, the system can be thrown off balance. We have seen the dramatic effects of pollution and ecological imbalance in nature, where everything has its purpose, down to the smallest insect that helps break down decaying protein and ready it for absorption back into the soil. When the balance of nature is upset, undesirable results occur.

Similarly, when our systems get thrown off balance by food impoverished of natural elements through refining processes, conditions arise which we find disturbing: such as overweight. This is not to say that all of our modern food processing techniques are to be condemned; but in too many cases, science has seen fit to try and improve on nature, with occasional unfortunate results.

Excessive food of any type can cause overweight, and rather than play around with diet pills without the benefit of medical guidance, I suggest that we pay more attention to the food we eat and include more *natural* foods in our diets.

What do I mean by *natural* foods? Just what the name implies: food as it comes from nature. Fruit allowed to ripen to maturity, thereby containing more of the vital elements, enzymes and nourishment that are destroyed, for example, when tomatoes are picked green and brought to maturity by chemical sprays and artificial means to add color. Vegetables grown and ripened naturally, then brought to market without any type of treatment to enhance appearance. Natural, not processed, cheeses. The list is almost endless, and is given in more detail further in this book.

With today's high prices, you will find that choosing natural foods can save money as well as improve your health and weight. Fresh brussels sprouts, carefully cooked and served with a natural cheese sauce, will work out to about half the cost of a similar dish prepared in a little aluminum foil pan, and sold frozen. You may spend a little more time preparing your meals, but is it not worth it—not only for health, but also to help get your weight back to its desired, normal level? Convenience foods may save time and effort, but at the expense of nutrition and calories, as well as your budget. So start thinking natural food and using more of it in your daily cooking. You'll be doing yourself and your family a favor.

Usually, basic natural foods are cheaper than processed, prepared foods, particularly those put out by an organization dedicated to weight control, whose recommended dishes appear slanted only towards those able to *afford* to lose weight! One frozen "meal" which sells for approximately 80 cents contains a small piece of fish and a vegetable; by preparing the identical items yourself, using fresh fish and natural vegetables, you could save yourself about 50 cents and have the advantage of eating food uncontaminated by the artificial additives and preservatives necessary to maintain the frozen item for weeks in the store.

Small frozen meat pies are another example

of convenience foods that may be filling and tasty, but not overly nourishing. With few exceptions, most brands of frozen meat pies contain approximately a dessert spoon of meat (not always tender or free from gristle), a similar amount of finely chopped potatoes and carrots, perhaps a few peas, and plenty of rich, thick gravy, encased in a pastry shell. While the pie may taste delicious, the actual food value is questionable. In addition, the amount of preservatives and flavor enhancers in frozen pies can often cause severe heartburn.

You have only to compare the price of plain frozen vegetables with those encased in plastic pouches and garnished with some type of thick sauce. The processed, packaged vegetables, sometimes called "exotic" or "international", may have an aura of glamor to them, but are far more expensive than the basic, natural items.

There has been a great deal of resistance among the general public towards natural foods, or organically grown fruits and vegetables, as they are sometimes called. I blame the dogmatic food faddists for this. Extremes are always dangerous in any activity, and including natural foods in your daily meals does not mean you'll have to switch to bowls of crushed nuts and dried alfalfa! With few exceptions, your menu will look very much the same as it does now; the difference will be felt and experienced in better health for your family—and the gradual adjustment to proper proportions of anyone who suffers from a weight problem.

Changing to natural foods does not mean a cataclysmic revolution in your kitchen or shopping schedules. It does not mean searching for a health food store, because many suitable items are available in your supermarket. Eating naturally *will* mean eliminating certain food items from your menu, plus a little more care in food preparation, but is this so much to ask of anyone who wants to get in shape—the right shape?

Eating natural foods does not mean your eating regimen will become unappealing. You will merely have to revise your food intake, substituting natural food for processed or prepared dishes, and watching what you eat. If you consider this tedious, think about it the next time you step on the scale!

This detailed explanation of the philosophy behind natural foods is predicated not only on my belief in eating properly, but in helping others *understand* why they should follow certain rules in selecting foodstuffs at the market. It is not enough to get directions and choose certain items because you've been told they're better for you. You have to be aware of *why* these items are better for you, and be able to look out for those products which contain potentially harmful additives. This takes some mental discipline.

Yet without this discipline and understanding, you're liable, after a week or two, to become careless and say to yourself, "What the hell, a piece of pie won't hurt." The fact remains: A piece of pie may well negate all the good you've done beforehand, especially if it's one of those prepared frozen pies, all ready to pop in the oven. I'm not against apple pie *per se,* provided it's made from scratch with fresh apples, unprocessed flour and acceptable ingredients. It's all that artifical gook that doesn't always sit well on the stomach!

Apple pie, naturally, brings up the matter of calories. You may have thought by now that all you have to do is eat natural foods and your weight will miraculously return to normal. Not so, unless you watch the quantity, and also count the calories. By this I do not mean a rigid calorie count on every single item; more people have given up diets because of being poor at mathematics! But a broad, overall assessment of your intake is essential, and this is dealt with in detail in a later chapter. Common sense should also come to your rescue. There are some people for whom one potato means an extra two inches on the waistline. If you know this, then obviously you don't eat potatoes, natural, processed, dehydrated or whatever!

Calories are calories, whether they come in natural or processed foods, so don't think you can overlook this important aspect of weight control. In a later section, I will be giving examples of diets for various persons in different occupations, men and women, taken from actual case histories of patients whom I have successfully treated for overweight. Many people consume between 5,000 and 6,000 calories daily, and then wonder why their bodies bloat. Through switching to the right natural foods, most people can eat well, have a good, tempting variety of food on the table, yet still lose weight by keeping the calories down to 1,000 to 1,600 a day. In some cases, where the individual is engaged in active work, the daily caloric intake can be as high as 2,000; but again, I stress that you will be giving your body a better chance to adjust and get back to normal by eliminating processed foods and all the artificial additives that only clutter up your metabolism. Knowing what food *is* and what it does for you will enable you to plan your menus with greater awareness of how a meal will affect your health and weight.

In the following chapter, we detail the basic breakdown of foods into their staple division; breads, meats, milk and milk products, fruits and vegetables. We discuss the content of food: protein, carbohydrates and fats, vitamins and minerals.

We give comparisons between commonly used food items and their counterpart in natural foods, together with a substitution table that will enable you to replace less desirable items with those that are better for you. And such substitutions do not sacrifice taste, appearance or appeal.

Briefly, I want you to feel as strongly as I do about the importance of natural foods—both for our general health and for helping control and adjust our weight.

Some of us, due to our occupations or life-styles, are unable to adhere to a specified diet, particularly one involving the use of natural foods. People who travel a great deal are particularly prone to weight problems because of the irregularity of meal times and having to eat in restaurants where the quality of food may be questionable.

For such people, I recommend the avoidance of obviously undesirable foods such as overly processed desserts and main dishes, and ordering instead plain meat, fish or poultry courses with plain vegetables or fresh salads and fresh fruit. And to insure an adequate supply of natural vitamins and minerals, there are food supplements, such as Nutrilite, which are not made chemically, but extracted from natural foods such as alfalfa, watercress, parsley, fish oils and yeast. The key to food supplements, as with food served on the table, is *natural*.

The following chapters illustrate how you can prepare some extremely appealing and exotic-looking dishes using natural foods, so that you will still get compliments on the appearance of your meals as well as the satisfaction· of knowing every morsel is contributing to your family's health and proper weight level.

Serving natural foods to your family will not only aid adult weight control and improve health generally, but will give your children a head start in health that will have lifetime benefits.

Natural foods might be called "normalizers" of weight; over and above this, they provide us with a greater chance of securing and maintaining the most priceless possession of all—good health.

Chapter One

The Food We Eat

Whether you have a weight problem or not, you should maintain a well-balanced daily intake of food to enable your body to operate at maximum efficiency. Just as your car coughs and sputters on inferior gasoline with a low octane rating, so do our bodies operate less effectively on foods that lack an adequate amount of essential nutrients: *protein, fats and carbohydrates, vitamins* and *minerals*. Knowing the purpose of these elements, and which food items contain the highest amounts, will help you plan your menu with an eye to health as well as to getting the most food value for your dollar.

Protein

Protein is the most important ingredient in any diet, because without a daily intake of it, the body cannot replace living cells. Protein forms the tissues, nerves, bones, hair, fingernails and the hemoglobin in the blood, and is therefore essential not only to health, but to life itself.

When protein enters the stomach in the form of food, it is broken down into amino acids which the body uses to form new tissue, or fresh protein. There are about 24 amino acids whose need has been established as vital to our health, more than half of which are synthesized by the body. The rest have to be provided in the daily diet, and include arginine, arpartic acid, cirruline, glutamic acid, glycine, hydroxyproline, hydroxyglutamic acid, norleucine, proline, serine and tyrosine.

The utilization of protein in the foods we eat is dependent upon the stomach acids. Those who take antacids regularly, such as bicarbonate of soda or Alka-Seltzer, may find temporary relief from the discomfort of over-eating, but at the same time, they are inhibiting the normal chemical action which enables protein to be absorbed and utilized. Rather than take antacids, one should limit the intake of food, particularly spicy dishes which can cause heartburn.

There are many sources of protein, the best one being meat or fish. Being similar to our own bodies, animal tissue breaks down into the proper proportion of amino acids which the body is able to absorb most efficiently. Because of this, meat and fish are the most important items in our diet, being not only the most complete form of protein, but the one most easily assimilated by our bodies.

There are those who claim we can get all the protein we need from vegetables, but the amount and proportion of amino acids obtained from vegetable protein is far less than from animal protein.

A totally strict vegetarian, therefore, runs the risk of a possible protein deficiency with a diet that excludes all meat or animal products such as eggs, milk or cheese.

Our bodies absorb 97 percent of meat protein, but only 85 percent of protein in cereals and fruits, and 78 percent in legumes. The daily requirement of protein is between 60 and 90 grams for women and 70 to 100 grams for men. This means we should include at least one serving of meat every day in our diet, a minimum of 3 ounces, which is really not very much. Weigh three ounces of ground meat on a postal scale and you'll be surprised at the quantity: far less than a normal size steak or a hamburger.

Although eating more protein than one normally needs does help to melt fat away, eating *only* protein would violate a basic rule of any diet: *balance*. Any excess protein that is ingested is converted into glucose and stored in the body. A balance between all the constituents in a good diet is the key to health and normal weight. The right quantity and quality of protein is vital, just as with other food constituents.

The following table gives a brief summary of some of the commonest foods and the number of grams of protein in 100 grams of the particular item in its most commonly used form:

Almonds	18.6
Apples	.2
Asparagus	2.2
Bacon	30.4

Beef: T-Bone Steak 19.5

      Hamburger 24.2

      Liver 26.4

Cola beverages 0

Bread: White enriched 8.7

      Wholewheat 10.8

Chocolate 4.2

Cashew Nuts 17.2

Cheese: Cottage 13.6

      Swiss 27.5

Eggs 12.9

Flounder 30.0

Gelatin 35.6

Ice Cream 4.5

Lentils: Raw 24.7

      Cooked 7.8

Lima Beans 7.6

Milk 3.5

Mussels 18.2

Orange 1.0

Peanuts 26.0

Peas 2.9

Rice: Brown 2.5

      White 2.0

Salmon 22.5

Soybeans: Raw 34.1

      Cooked 11.0

Spaghetti 5.0

Sugars 0

Sunflower seeds 24

Tuna (canned) 24.2

Vegetable juice 9

Yogurt 3.0

You can supplement your meals with protein-rich snacks that will provide sustenance without excessive calories: hard-boiled eggs; deviled eggs made with your favorite spice or herbs; wedges of natural hard cheese; a slice of cooked meat, such as turkey, chicken, duck or beef; cottage cheese, again herbed to your taste if desired; sunflower or pumpkin seeds; raw nuts; sardines, tuna fish or salmon; a gelatin salad, with or without fruit or vegetables. These items all fit into the "six-small-snacks-a-day" regimen described in a later chapter.

You may have noticed that in the above list, under "cheese", only "cottage" and "Swiss" were mentioned. We are pointing the way back to nattural foods rather than artificial; in other words, cottage cheese and Swiss cheese are preferred over processed cheese, both from a nutritional standpoint as well as taste and bodily benefit. Whenever possible, substitution can help bring natural goodness back into your menu.

Fats

Protein forms the tissues of the body, but our energy comes from fats (and carbohydrates), fast sources of fuel to keep us going. Some people believe that eliminating fat from the diet will take care of excess poundage. Not so! Fats should make up 25 percent of our diet, but most Americans eat as much as 40 percent fat in the varied assortment of goodies they shovel into their stomachs each day; and then they wonder why they are overweight!

Fats are as essential to our well-being as protein; for without them, the fat-soluble vitamins A, D, E and K, could not be absorbed, and we would also miss out on Vitamin F, the unsaturated fatty acids. The difficulty with identifying fatty items in the diet lies in not realizing that all fatty foods do not *look* fatty! Butter, margarine and oils are simple to spot, but do you realize that milk, cheese, eggs, peanut butter, bologna, olives and avocados all have at least one third fat in their innocent looking exteriors? Similarly, even lean steak or fillet contains fat, which is why for dieters, we recommend whitefish over steak as a source of low-fat protein.

Eaten together with protein, fat can be fully utilized by the body mechanism, burning properly like the fuel in a car when the mixture is right. If the body supply of protein is insufficient, fat will not be burned so rapidly, another reason we should eat more whitefish and eggs than steak. Fats also contain many substances essential to balanced nutrition, such as linoleic acid, and three fatty acids necessary for the right use and absorption of saturated fats and cholesterol. Without linoleic, linolenic and arachidonic acids in the diet, cholesterol can build up and result in clogged arteries and possible heart attacks.

Carbohydrates

Carbohydrates come in various forms: starches, sugars, dextrins, celluloses, pectins and gums, and apart from providing energy and bulk, they provide some essential vitamins and minerals that the body needs for its metabolic processes. Bread provides carbohydrates, as well as protein, calcium, phosphorous, iron, sodium, potassium, Vitamin A, some of the B complex vitamins, and Vitamin C. Potatoes provide even more Vitamin C and most of the essential minerals.

Carbohydrates have achieved somewhat of a bad name among dieters, but, in actuality, only the highly refined food items, such as sugar, fall into this category. Sugar and alcohol have no value other than supplying energy, but not always in the most beneficial manner. Normally, starches and carbohydrates are converted into sugar by the normal body functions. Putting refined sugar into our stomachs is giving our metabolism a concentrated "shot" which it was not originally meant to handle. This causes the pancreas to secrete extra amounts of insulin, lowering the level of blood-sugar; after the initial surge of energy from the sugar, we get a let-down because of the extra insulin. The resulting tiredness creates a demand for more sugar for more energy, creating a never-ending up-and-down cycle. Refined sugar not only upsets the blood-suger balance but also contributes largely to tooth decay. Candy and soft drinks may be great taste-treats, but do little for nutrition and dental health; our children would be better off eating fresh fruits and nuts instead.

As with fats, excessive carbohydrates in the diet are a major cause of overweight today. They are essential to a balanced menu, but only in the right proportions, and preferably from natural sources.

Vitamins

For all the thousands of parts that make up an automobile engine, plus the essential fuel, a car would remain stationary if there were no spark to ignite the gasoline and keep things moving; similarly, in the human body, vitamins provide the spark that helps our metabolism assimilate the food we eat, changing sugars and fats into energy, and breaking down protein into amino acids for growth and building up the protein muscle mass. These minute chemical substances are essential to regulate our body mechanism, and they all work together, each in its own way and in its required amount, in the interests of nutrition and health. Vitamins are key factors in our food absorption and bodily well-being. Deficiencies in certain vitamins can cause a chain reaction of ill effect, just as too much of one vitamin can destroy the effectiveness of another.

However, due to our life-style and eating habits, not everybody gets sufficient vitamins in the diet, so balanced natural food supplements can be most beneficial, even with a diet of natural foods; supplements are particularly advisable for those on diets with a restricted intake of food.

Vitamin A: Being a fat soluble substance, Vitamin A is stored in the body. Our natural supply of this vitamin can be diminished by taking laxatives containing mineral oil.

The minimum daily requirement is 400 International Units, an amount usually included in the average intake of protein foods rich in Vitamin A.

Some nutrition experts claim that markedly excessive use of Vitamin A can be toxic and cause a wide variety of unpleasant symptoms from headaches and blurred vision to painful joints.

In its correct amount, Vitamin A contributes to the health of the linings of all body organs, bones and tooth enamel, and one of its functions is to reduce the level of cholesterol in the blood. A deficiency of Vitamin A produces night blindness, dry skin and hair, and gallstones.

Among the richest sources of Vitamin A is casaba melon, with 100,000 International Units per 100 grams, and liver, with 53,400 units per 100 grams. Other foods high in Vitamin A are carrots, red peppers, sweet potatoes, parsley and watercress, collards, chicken livers and egg yolks. Carotene, a substance found in green and yellow vegetables, is converted by the body into Vitamin A, supplementing that obtained from meat and fish protein.

Vitamin B Complex: The B complex, as suggested by its name, is a complex structure of substances which depend upon each other for the proper working of each particular vitamin. A deficiency of one will result in a mass deficiency, and an excess of one will likewise cause adverse reaction among the other members of the B family. They are all water soluble compounds and include: Thiamine (Vitamin B1 and Aneurine), Riboflavin (Vitamin B2 and Vitamin G), Niacin (Nicotinic Acid), Pyridoxin (Pyridoxin Hydrochloride, B6), Pantothenic Acid, Biotin (Vitamin H and R), Folic Acid, Cobalamin (B12), Inositol, Choline, Para-Aminobenzoic Acid (Citrovorum), Vitamin B13, Vitamin B14.

Thiamine (Vitamin B1): Thiamine is important for physical and mental energy, as it acts upon starches and sugars, changing them into energy. Deficiency can cause tiredness, weakness and shortness of breath, which in turn can lead to irritability and depression and a host of nervous disorders.

Being water-soluble, thiamine is eliminated in the body by excessive alcohol, alkalizers and sugar. This vitamin is also destroyed by heat through over-cooking, another reason for watching the clock after you put vegetables on the stove. Cooking anything too long is only wasting fuel and short-changing your family on food value.

A good natural source of thiamine is wheat germ, as well as brewer's yeast, which has a particularly high content (15.61 milligrams per 100 grams).

Brewer's yeast is often prescribed for people with nervous complaints, another example of natural foods providing the nutrients we need to keep *naturally* healthy. The minimum daily requirement of thiamine has been set at 2 milligrams, or approximately the amount you would get in 100 grams of rice bran.

Riboflavin (Vitamin B2): Like B1, this vitamin helps convert starches and sugars into energy, as well as helping maintain bodily resistance to disease, working with thiamine, pantothenic acid and Vitamin A in the various body functions. A lack of riboflavin can result in problems affecting the eyes, including general soreness and cloudy vision.

The minimum daily requirement is 3 milligrams. Good sources of Vitamin B2 are beef liver, chicken liver, sesame seeds and brewer's yeast.

Niacin (Nicotinic Acid): Niacin works with riboflavin in converting starches and sugars into energy, and like Vitamin A, it can diminish the cholesterol in the bloodstream.

A niacin deficiency causes pellagra, and also a variety of nervous disorders.

The minimum daily requirement is 24 milligrams. Foods high in niacin include bran, brewer's yeast, chicken liver, dried malt, peaches, peppers, and salmon.

Pyridoxin (Vitamin B6): This vitamin works on the conversion of protein, and helps in the utilization of fats and formation of blood. Pyridoxin is of benefit to people with ailments and to those suffering from lack of muscular control due to palsy and Parkinson's disease.

Deficiency of this vitamin is evidenced by lack of nerve control, sickness and dizziness, and some skin ailments.

The minimum daily requirement has not been specifically determined, though estimated at 1 to 2 milligrams. Vitamin B6 is found in eggs, fish, milk, nuts, seeds, rice polishings, whole-wheat, blackstrap molasses, animal entrails and brewer's yeast.

Cobalamin (Vitamin B12): Cobalamin acts in the formation of blood cells, and, as such, has been a literal life-saver for those suffering from pernicious anemia. Deficiency of cobalamin brings about malformation of the bone marrow.

The minimum daily requirement is unknown, but estimated at 1 microgram. The best sources of this vitamin are also the best sources of protein, especially liver and kidneys.

Folic Acid (Vitamin M): Like cobalamin, folic acid helps in the formation of red blood cells. Cells cannot divide without it being present in the system. Folic acid works in conjunction with cobalamin in the treatment of pernicious anema, leukemia and several forms of cancer.

Folic acid is found chiefly in leafy vegetables, and is destroyed by exposure to light and heat, another reason to avoid overcooking green vegetables. This vitamin is also present in whole

31

wheat and, in abundant amounts, in brewer's yeast, liver, heart, brains and kidneys. The minimum daily requirement has not been established.

Cholin: Cholin affects the distribution of fats throughout the body and helps the gallbladder operate efficiently. A deficiency of cholin causes an accumulation of fats in the liver.

The daily requirements have been set at 50 milligrams per kilo of body weight.

Cholin is found in brain, tongue, root vegetables, brewer's yeast, liver and wheat germ, with a high proportion in egg yolk.

Pantothenic Acid: This substance is another example of the B-complex vitamins working together, for without pantothenic acid, cholin is unable to perform its function properly. In addition, pantothenic acid helps forestall symptoms of old age, and is of great value in helping the body handle toxic substances such as DDT, cortisone, streptomycin; it is also given to people suffering from mental stress. No minimum daily requirement has been established.

Pantothenic acid is present in large quantities in liver, egg yolk and brewer's yeast, as well as heart, brain, mushrooms, broccoli, peas, peanuts and soybeans.

Biotin (Vitamin H): Soluble in alcohol as well as water, biotin is essential for the growth of yeast fungi and bacteria which are all part of the human metabolism. The function of biotin is similar to pantothenic acid, helping in the assimilation and digestion of fats in the body. Deficiency of biotin can result in dermatitis and mental depression.

The highest concentration of biotin is in brewer's yeast, veal, cauliflower, liver and egg yolk.

Inositol: This substance is present in all the cells of the body, and works with cholin and Vitamin A in controlling the cholesterol level in the blood. Inositol also aids the absorption of Vitamin E. Little is known about its actual function, and no minimum daily requirement has been set. Inositol is present in brewer's yeast, brains, heart, liver, lima beans, peas and wheat germ.

Para-Aminobenzoic Acid (PABA): This element works with folic acid in many of the same functions, and together with cholin, inositol and pantothenic acid, it has helped maintain hair color, preventing grayness. No minimum daily requirement has been established.

PABA is found in brewer's yeast, liver, blackstrap molasses and whole grains.

This concludes the list of vitamins and elements generally called the B-complex, because, as we have seen, they work together and depend on each other for the proper chemical reaction within the body and the maintenance of health.

Vitamin C (Ascorbic Acid): Vitamin C is essential in our daily diet as this is one substance which cannot be synthesized by the body (as with higher plants and most animals) nor can it be stored in the tissues. The vitamin is very unstable, evaporating on exposure to light. The daily glass of fresh, pure orange juice is more than a tasty breakfast drink; it is an essential supplement in that well-balanced diet that is so important for our health.

Vitamin C works with minerals in the formation of bones and teeth; it helps the body utilize iron; it regulates cholesterol in the blood and, like pantothenic acid, helps combat the toxic effects of chemical additives that may find their

33

way into our food. Vitamin C also has anti-histaminic properties, making it a popular remedy for the common cold, though it should not be looked upon as a cure, no matter how it may appear to help.

Deficiency of Vitamin C leads to bad teeth and gums, brittle bones, kidney stones, fatigue, sterility and weakness. Extreme lack causes scurvy, a rare skin disease today, but common years ago among sailors who undertook long voyages without fresh vegetables.

The minimum daily requirement is between 75 and 100 milligrams, but no untoward effects have been noted from far higher dosages.

Vitamin C is found almost entirely in fresh fruit and vegetables, with especially high amounts in currants, guavas, parsley and red peppers.

Smokers are particularly advised to take a good daily ration of Vitamin C, as one cigarette neutralizes 25 milligrams of this vitamin, which is also destroyed by aspirin and by stress.

Vitamin D: Commonly called "the sunshine vitamin," Vitamin D is produced by the body through exposure to sunlight, but can also be ingested by eating fish, butter, eggs, milk and sunflower seeds, as well as concentrated natural cod-liver oil.

Vitamin D operates in close association with Vitamin A in the absorption of calcium and phosphorous in the body, and is therefore essential for the proper growth of teeth and bones, and especially important for women during pregnancy and lactation.

Deficiency of Vitamin D results in the improper utilization of sugar, with resultant fatigue and nervousness; defective teeth and bone structure follow a lack of Vitamin D in the diet and in extreme cases, rickets.

Vitamin E (Tocopherol): Vitamin E works as a tissue builder, and seems to help prevent ugly scar tissue. A fat soluble vitamin, tocopherol works with other vitamins as a detoxifier and has an ability to conserve oxygen.

The minimum daily requirement has been set at 30 International Units, and natural Vitamin E possesses greater potency than synthetic. Wheat germ and vegetable oils are the best sources.

Vitamin F: Vitamin F is a term given unsaturated fatty acids, which help in the absorption of fat soluble vitamins A, D, E and K. The proper functioning of the thyroid gland and the reproductive organs is affected by the unsaturated fatty acids.

Deficiency in Vitamin F shows up in brittle, dull hair and nails, and in dry skin. Vegetable and seed oils, and whole grains are good sources of Vitamin F.

Vitamin K: Vitamin K promotes blood clotting by increasing the prothrombin content of the blood.

Deficiency results in abnormal bleeding and insufficient clotting. Vitamin K can be synthesized by bacteria in the body, and is found in green vegetables, tomatoes, strawberries, rose hips and liver.

Vitamin P (Bioflavanoids): This water soluble vitamin is found in citrus fruits, rose hips and paprika, and helps maintain the resistance of cell and capillary walls. Deficiency of Vitamin P leads to subcutaneous bleeding. As this vitamin is always found in conjunction with Vitamin C, the two act together; an adequate daily intake of Vitamin C will insure sufficient Vitamin P as well, though a minimum daily requirement has not been determined. Acerola (Caribbean cherries) is among the highest natural sources of these vitamins.

Minerals

The presence of vitamins in the diet is vital to health; so also with minerals, which interact with vitamins in the metabolic function of digestion, helping break down protein into amino acids, as well as being essential to the maintenance of tissue. Minerals help maintain the proper water balance in the body, and help preserve the alkaline balance in blood and tissue. Some minerals form a basic part of the body structure, such as calcium, which forms 2 percent of body weight in bones and teeth. Like vitamins, minerals are utilized in very small amounts, but nevertheless are important in the healthy functioning of all parts of the body.

Calcium: Calcium is found abundantly in milk and certain milk products, but is also present in most foods in minute quantities. Calcium works closely with phosphorous, the proper balance of both minerals being vital to their being fully utilized. Deficiency in calcium results in cramps, nervous tension, rapid heartbeat, tooth decay, brittle bones and premature aging. The minimum daily requirement for men and women is 800 milligrams: for children and pregnant women, 1200 milligrams. Chocolate and cocoa inhibit the absorption of calcium, another reason (apart from tooth decay) to limit a child's intake of these sweets.

Good sources of calcium are milk and milk products, especially Parmesan, Swiss and cheddar cheese; blackstrap molasses and kelp.

Phosphorous: Phosphorous is found in all living human tissue and works with calcium in the formation of bones and teeth. Phosphorous is necessary in the process that converts protein into amino acids and fats and carbohydrates into energy, and as such is essential to human nutrition. Phosphorous and calcium work together with Vitamin D, these three substances being dependent upon each other for assimilation into the system.

The highest proportion of phophorous in food is found in whole grains, soybeans, cranberries and poultry.

Iron: Being important in conveying oxygen to blood cells, iron is vital to the diet. Although present in most foods, iron is needed in supplemental form by many people. Deficiency of iron or secondary anemia results in fatigue and lowered resisitance to disease.

The minimum daily requirement is 12 milligrams for men and 15 milligrams for children, young people and pregnant women. A good supply of iron is present in legumes, green vegetables, cereals, nuts and milk.

Copper: Helping in the assimilation of Vitamin C and iron, copper also works to produce red blood cells by the bone marrow.

Together with iron and iodine, copper helps maintain healthy reproductive organs. Deficiency of copper results in chronic weakness, anemia and difficulty in breathing.

Magnesium: Roughly 70 percent of the magnesium in the human body is present in the bones, with the rest distributed in blood and tissue. It is helpful in normal muscular activity, as well as in working with Vitamin B6 as a natural tranquilizer. A component of chlorophyll, magnesium starts certain chemical actions in the body and helps with the enzyme action of building protein. An example of the independence of all vitamins and minerals in our diet, magnesium works with the enzyme action involving calcium and phosphorous. Without magnesium, the bones suffer from calcification.

Magnesium is found in green leaves, seeds and nuts.

Zinc: Zinc is present in all body tissue, mostly in the pancreas, where it is concerned with the output of insulin, as well as its proper utilization. Zinc is involved in the chemical reactions of thiamine and pyrodoxin, and functions as a catalyst in the production of energy.

Potassium: Together with sodium and chlorine, potassium is necessary for the maintenance of body fluids, and is important in the proper functioning of the nervous and cardiac systems.

Deficiency in potassium slows down normal body growth and contributes to constipation and nervousness. Present in most foods, potassium is found in greatest quantity in green vegetables.

Sodium Chloride: Both sodium and chlorine are found in common salt (sodium chloride). These two elements help control body fluids. Salt is essential to our body functions, as the chlorine in it helps in the formation of hydrochloric acid in the stomach which helps break down food. Lack of salt can cause lassitude and exhaustion, the reason people sometimes take salt pills during very hot weather when too much salt is lost through perspiration. Beets, leafy green vegetables, radishes and olives provide extra sources of chlorine.

Iodine: Iodine is needed for the proper functioning of the thyroid gland. Although only a minute amount of iodine is needed, it is vital to our health, working with the thyroid in maintaining weight, health and mental stability.

Deficiency of iodine in the system leads to goiter, with overweight, slow reactions and lowered mentality.

Most foods that come from the sea are rich in iodine, especially dulse and kelp and, of course, all seafoods and shellfish.

Trace Minerals: Additional minerals significant to our health include aluminum, boron, bromine, cobalt, fluorine, manganese, nickel, silver, silicon and sulphur. These all affect the composition of the blood and help regulate the function of the tissues.

As with many of the vitamins, minerals are found most abundantly in natural foods, freshly picked and not overcooked. The best way to get your minimum daily requirements of all vitamins and minerals is to insure you get an adequate supply of food, grown the way nature intended, with a minimum of refining or processing. It's an old cliché, but still true: We are what we eat. And the more natural food we include in our diet, the more naturally healthy our bodies will be— and the better chance we give ourselves to achieve and maintain a proper weight level.

Chapter Two

Natural or Processed Food?

Health foods have proven to be more than a passing fad. Have you checked the newest items on the shelves at the market? There is a definite trend back to nature, with many cereal manufacturers bringing out "natural" cereals; in their commercials on television, stress is placed upon the lack of artificial additives or preservatives.

This is more than a gimmick to attract extra sales; the food manufacturers have realized that people are becoming aware once again of the value of natural foods—of the grains as they come from the fields, rich with nutritive value and bursting with goodness, the vitamins and minerals intact, ready to go to work in the body the way they were intended.

So broadly speaking, we advocate your buying natural and cooking natural—that is, sticking to the basics rather than the more esoteric dishes that are not always advisable for people with weight problems. Again we stress that this does not mean switching to a menu that lacks eye or taste appeal, as you will see when you get to later chapters dealing with cooking and recipes.

We also are not intending to discredit the packaged dishes. We are merely pointing out that you can do your health a lot more good (and also ease your food budget!) by deciding to prepare from scratch, using natural foods at every opportunity.

Your supermarket abounds with items that fit into a natural diet. Take the milk product counter for example: There is a staggering array of cheeses, but in addition to the processed cheese, there is natural cheese. It may not be sliced and individually wrapped in plastic (a wonderful convenience, admittedly) but don't forget you pay for that feature, both in food value and cost of the actual item. A block of natural cheese will be cheaper and give you a higher percentage of nutritional value. And perhaps most importantly: It will *taste* better!

Let's talk about vegetables; both fresh and frozen. We have nothing against frozen vegetables; in fact, they are often a better buy because of lack of waste and prime quality. We do quibble at the "exotic" assortments, usually in plastic pouches with sauces added, mainly because you can put your own assortment together from the basic vegetables themselves, and add your own sauce, freshly prepared with more wholesome ingredients—*and* at half the price! Using natural, or organically grown, items gives you the added bonus of fresher tasting, more nutritive dishes, too. There is also the advantage of having none of the chemical preservatives needed to keep the items salable in the store, and each unnecessary chemical you keep out of your body, the further ahead you are towards *natural* health!

Tomatoes are a prime example of how much better the natural product is over the artificial: On your produce counter, you have seen vine-ripened tomatoes, usually loose, by the pound and you have seen the packaged kind, usually four or six in a plastic container, priced by the container. Do we have to tell you which tastes better? The vine-ripened, naturally, because being allowed to ripen on the vine, they contain all the enzymes, vitamins and minerals that nature puts there, whereas the packaged variety are often picked green, then artificially brought to maturity through chemical sprays and light; this variety is not nearly as tasty and juicy, nor is there the same nutritive value.

So many of the food items we use every day are processed to such an extent that much of the natural goodness has been removed.

Many of the natural food faddists claim that any food that is *not* natural (i.e., processed in some fashion) is not good for one. This is ridiculous, as are most extreme viewpoints. Better to adopt the attitude that where naural foods can be substituted for a processed product, you will be better off, nutrition-wise, to go the natural route; also, you will be better off budget-wise. Processed foods cost more, and the deterioration of vitamins and minerals through the processing makes them an even less appealing value for the money, no matter how appealing they look and taste.

This book is concerned mainly with weight problems and from this standpoint, processed foods invariably are hazardous, containing too many calories and insufficient natural nutrients. So our constant stressing of natural foods over processed stems from our desire to point out the foods that are best for your weight control, as well as for your general health.

Merely switching to natural foods without counting calories is not going to do the trick, even though you will benefit in general health. Calories are calories, no matter what form they take; so you still have to limit your intake of natural foods if you intend to lose weight. However, smaller quantities of natural foods enable you to gain in nutrition and overall health at the same time as you lose those unwanted pounds. The minimum daily requirements of protein, fats, carbohydrates, vitamins and minerals must still be met even by dieters, otherwise general health is impaired. A restricted diet of processed foods can sometimes mean a hazardous lack of essential nutrients, making the addition of nutritional supplements in pill form often essential; with natural foods, you can get more of the vital elements you need, and no potentially harmful chemical additives are introduced into your system.

So let's start with your basic shopping list, presuming at this point that you are eager to stock your shelves with more natural food items in preparation for switching to a natural diet to improve your health as well as to lose (or gain) weight. Dieting has, quite naturally, come to mean losing rather than gaining weight, because most Americans suffer from overweight, thanks to giving in to temptation when those fabulous processed foods appear on the table! In a recent national survey, 60 percent of men and women admitted they felt they could lose weight to advantage. The fantastic sale of diet books also attests to the fact that we, as a nation, are concerned about staying slender; we talk a lot about it, but how many really *do* something about it?

We hope that by switching to natural foods, you will be taking the first step towards making health and a normal weight a natural part of your life, as it should be.

Back to the shopping list: There are many items you now use which can be replaced with natural food items, doing the same job, but giving additional benefits in nutritive value. Also, by knowing what to avoid and what to look for, you can improve the quality of those items available to you—not all of us have access to naturally produced meat, eggs and cheese, yet we can watch for indications of freshness in the market that will mean more flavor and vitamin content.

Take eggs for a start: If you cannot locate a source for fresh, fertile, farm-produced eggs, which would be our recommendation, then try for a store that sells eggs with dated cartons. The nutritive value of eggs deteriorates at room temperature and exposure to light; eggs should be refrigerated in their original cartons, kept closed. The open shelves in the refrigerator door may be convenient, but lead to faster loss of quality. How can you tell if an egg is fresh? By its ability to stand up when opened: If the white runs and the yolk breaks, you have old stock. A fresh egg will sit in the pan, firm, the yolk nicely rounded above the white, which does not run. You'll also be ahead in value by buying the largest size eggs you can get. Small eggs are usually only about 20 cents to 30 cents a dozen less than extra-large. You would use two small eggs to one extra large, so obviously it is cheaper to buy the larger size.

As for milk, some stores stock natural, raw milk (meaning not pasteurized) which is preferable, provided it comes from healthy, inspected cows and a sanitary source. Pasteurization has admittedly helped cut down on disease-carrying milk, but the process destroys a percentage of the natural goodness and vitamins.

While some dairies offer a "Vitamin D enriched" milk, one can obtain all the Vitamin D needed from other sources, making the extra cost of "enriched" milk unnecessary. Regular homogenized, pasteurized milk sells for less than the enriched and fulfills the requirements for milk in the diet, although raw milk is still the best type to get. Low fat milk is better for dieters, but we recommend skim milk over all other types. For those who have trouble digesting milk, there are the fermented milk products, such as buttermilk, kumiss, kefir, and yogurt. Touted on television as "energy foods", these actually provide protein as well as natural enzymes, vitamins and minerals that are recommended additions to any diet, particularly as a between-meal snack that is high in nourishment and low in calories. These items are easier to digest than plain milk.

On cheeses, cheddar, Swiss and Parmesan are high in nutritive value, but, again, look for the natural product rather than the processed. Your market should stock both, and while the processed is often more attractively packaged and conveniently wrapped in individual slices, the bulk natural cheese is cheaper and better for you. With

45

cottage cheese, check the date on the package, as this item tends to spoil quickly. An alternative to cottage cheese is ricotta, a similar, soft cheese with a creamier taste and usually with less salt added. Cream cheese should also be checked for freshness, and buying it in bulk (the natural, rather than packaged type) gives you an edge in price and in purity.

On grains: Flour and bread has come under the constant condemnation of food faddists, and not without good reason. But if you prefer not to bake your own bread from natural whole wheat, freshly stone ground, look for the whole wheat variety in the store and avoid the overly processed white breads. Some smaller bakeries supply authentic "home-baked" bread, minus the chemical additives or preservatives that the larger mass-produced products contain. Such breads are worth looking for and paying a little more for, too. Many people are able to "wean" themselves from the taste of white, processed bread by gradually moving over to the natural product, using a slice of white and a slice of whole wheat for a sandwich, then after a few days, eliminating the white altogether. In reality, whole wheat bread is far tastier.

In your baking, generally select whole wheat flour over white flour. Again, if the taste factor intrudes on your enjoyment, use half white, and half whole wheat, gradually moving over completely to whole wheat as you become accustomed to the flavor.

White rice, while attractive in appearance, lacks any great specific taste unless perked up with gravy or sauce. In contrast, brown rice has a distinctive taste and is rich in natural nutrients. We suggest your reaching for the brown rice next time. Cooking it with beef or chicken bouillon instead of plain water and adding half a cup of pitted black olives and a half cup of sliced fresh mushrooms will give you a gourmet dish to tempt any palate, as well as a dish rich in the natural food elements missing in plain white rice.

Rice has several by-products that are excellent additions to your supply of staples: *rice bran,* which consists of the outer layers of bran from brown rice, a valuable source of nutrients and excellent for adding to breads, cookies and cereals; *rice flour,* in reality ground brown rice, a good flavor addition to other flours for baking; *rice grits,* coarsely cracked brown rice, an excellent addition to soups, stews and casseroles.

Barley comes pearled or polished, meaning stripped of some valuable food value. Buy the hulled whole grain barley, which can be used as a rice substitute, as well as in soups, stews and casseroles. *Barley flour* is barley grain that is ground, and adds nutrition and flavor to other flours for baking; however, lacking gluten (which is what makes bread hold together) it cannot be used exclusively for baking, but only in conjunction with other flours. Barley grits are also excellent for soups. Another good rice substitute (as well as a natural cereal) is buckwheat, whole grain hulled. Buckwheat flour can also be added to other flours for baking. Buckwheat pancakes are especially tasty as well as nutritious.

On oils and fats: The best butter to put on your table is freshly churned sweet cream; check the date on the package to insure freshness. However, for dieters we recommend margarine (corn oil, polyunsaturated) instead of butter.

For cooking and salad oils, there is a wide variety from which to choose: corn, olive, peanut, safflower, sesame, soybean and sunflower are all good, containing the three essential fatty acids (linoleic, linolenic, and arachidonic) as well as being high in unsaturated fats. To distinguish between fats and oils, remember the following: At room temperature, a solid item is considered a *fat;* if it is liquid, then it is an oil. The temperature naturally determines the condition, as warming lard (a fat) can turn it into a liquid (oil); some oils turn into fats when the temperature is lowered. The degree of liquid or solid depends on the saturation of fatty acids. The more solid they are, the higher the saturation. As a general rule, vegetable oils are highly unsaturated, while animal fats are highly saturated. Some people are also under the misconception that we should avoid all fats when dieting; one may have to *cut down,* but the body still needs its essential fatty acids to complete the normal nutritional requirements of any diet.

A good way to eliminate excess fat from the diet is to use lecithin to prevent eggs from sticking in the pan. If flavor is desired, a small amount of margarine may be used, not as much as you would normally use for frying, but just enough to give flavor to the eggs, depending on your particular preference.

Sugar is used in many dishes as well as for sweetening drinks. You can substitute for sugar with many natural sweeteners, such as blackstrap molasses, carob powder, carob syrup, date sugar, honey, malt, maple sugar, maple syrup, molasses and sorghum.

Blackstrap molasses is nutritionally rich, but because of its taste, should be used in conjunction with molasses or honey. Carob powder is obtained from the carob pod, and comes either plain or toasted. Toasted carob is similar to chocolate in flavor, but lacks the high fat content of chocolate, as well as having no stimulants. (Chocolate contains theobromine, a stimulant similar to caffeine, and is also not recommended for people suffering from migraine). Carob syrup is condensed from carob, and is a good natural sweetener. Date sugar is made from dried, ground dates, and is very good on cereal as well as in baking. Honey needs no explanation, other than to reiterate again its superb natural qualities of high nutrition, plus a pleasant variety of flavors depending on the type. Malt is a syrup made from germinated barley; it is good for baking and is somewhat less sweet than most natural sweeteners. Malt is especially palatable in milk drinks (the traditional soda fountain specialty: chocolate malt!). Maple syrup should be 100 percent pure, not the processed type. Maple sugar (which comes from maple syrup) is light brown, and with its tasty maple flavor, good in cooking and on cereals. Molasses should be the dark, unsulfured type. Sorghum is a natural sweetener made from grain, grown very much like corn. All these natural sweeteners are more potent than plain sugar and should be used sparingly, especially if you are unused to the taste. Experimenting with quantities will help you arrive at the right proportions to suit you. Although better nutritionally for you than refined sugars, natural sweeteners are all carbohydrates and should not be eaten excessively; and don't forget to include these in your calorie and carbohydrate count.

On meats: If you can locate a source for organically raised meat, meaning no feed concentrates, hormones or tranquilizers are fed to the animals, you'll be that much ahead in serving pure, natural meats to your family. However, as these are quite the exception, you will merely have to rely on your local supplier (butcher shop or supermarket) and follow these pointers: Have all visible fat trimmed away and have any hamburger ground freshly to your order. Do not buy the ready-ground variety, as this is high in fat content and often has filler in the form of meat scraps. You will get better value by purchasing chuck or round steak and having the butcher grind it while you wait, cutting off all fat beforehand. If you wish to stretch it yourself, you may add some of the various types of natural grains described earlier, adding protein, minerals and vitamins as well as the extra bulk.

Most often flour has been used as a thickener for soups and gravies, but you will find a wide choice of natural items that will be preferable: agar-agar, which is a sea vegetable similar to plain gelatin and excellent for thickening juices; arrow-root starch, which is used instead of white flour; plain gelatin (not Jell-O!), which needs no explanation; potato or tapioca starch or unbleached flour, all of which give you natural goodness plus thickening qualities.

You have probably noticed in the preceding chapter that brewer's yeast comes up in many areas as a prime source of the B-complex vitamins and protein. While many people take brewer's yeast, either in powder or tablet form, as a dietary supplement, you can also add it to your cooking routine. Since the taste is often pungent at first, you should start by adding only small amounts to fruit juices, soups, casseroles and batters. Brewer's yeast not only adds valuable nutrition to your meals, but a new and provocative flavor to many old dishes.

There are other valuable natural food additions that contribute vitamins and minerals to your food. *Kelp,* a seaweed which can be used as a seasoning, comes in granules or powder and is rich in minerals, vitamins and trace elements. Similar to kelp is *dulse,* also a seaweed and often eaten on the East Coast like candy. *Miso,* a protein made from soy beans, is good in soups and stews, added after cooking. *Sea salt* is richer in mineral content than the regular refined table salt. *Sunflower* and *sesame seeds* are good in baking and desserts. *Soy grits,* made from the cracked soy bean and containing more than twice the protein of meat, are good for adding to the ground meat in meat loaves and casseroles. *Wheat germ,* rich in protein and minerals, is good for adding to casseroles and cereals and for rolling meat and poultry in before cooking.

Sprouts, too, are excellent additions to any diet. Anyone who has ever partaken of Chinese food will know about bean sprouts, a staple in Chinese vegetables. Crisp, tasty and brimming with vitamins, sprouts need not be limited to Chinese cooking. Some people may feel that with an adequate daily intake of fresh, green vegetables, why bother with sprouts?

The reason stems from the vital nutrients present in sprouts. The majority of seeds, beans or grain will automatically increase their food content two or three times when sprouted: triple the vitamins, minerals and protein. For soups, salads and vegetable entrees, sprouts are highly recommended and are simple to grow.

The most popular are alfalfa, sunflower, fenu-greek, lentils, peas, mung beans, string beans, soy-beans, wheat and rye grains. Place a small quantity in a glass jar, cover with water and place a piece of cheese cloth over the top, holding this in place with a rubber band. Allow to stand over-night, then pour off the water in the morning, allowing fresh water to enter through the cheese cloth and rinse off the seeds, then draining it up-side-down, leaving the seeds moist but not stand-ing in water (otherwise they may rot). Place the glass jar in a dark, ventilated cupboard, and rinse morning and night; in three or four days, you should have sprouts the right size for eating. Sprouts may also be cultivated in the light; al-falfa, in particular, develops more chorophyll and better flavor this way. Soybeans, however, do bet-ter in the dark. A word of warning: Never eat potato sprouts, as these are poisonous. All other sprouts, however, provide a tasty addition to sal-ads, as well as to soups, stews, casseroles, scrambled eggs and on sandwiches, in place of lettuce. A fruit salad garnished with sprouts and yogurt is particularly delicious and nourishing.

Sprouts should be eaten daily, just like any other green vegetable, and, as such, you should rotate your crop, having three jars going, starting each a day apart. Sprouts are ready for use when 1/4" to 2" long, depending on the seed used. Sun-flowers, for example, are ideal when only 1/4" in length, but mung beans should be 2" to 3" long before using. Experimentation will be the best way to determine when your crop is ready for the table.

Some people are of the opinion that switching to natural foods means a drastic change in the

52

family eating habits. There are, admittedly, those who become fanatical on the subject, and many of the organic food books today give the impression that if you don't eat organically, you're liable to die from chemical poisoning before you're fifty! Which is, of course, ridiculous. However, it cannot be denied that the elimination of certain overly processed food items from the diet will benefit one's health; but this should not give you the idea that most of the products on the shelves should be avoided.

We advise a gradual change, for your family's sake. As we stress later on, the psychological attitudes towards dieting (or just plain eating) affect our metabolic responses and our reaction to food. Being such creatures of habit, we can sometimes nurture a resistance to change, particularly in regard to certain foods of which we have become particularly fond. There is a happy medium in everything, and we hope to arouse in you the realization that eating more natural foods, and less of the artificial, processed products, will bring about a general improvement in health, as well as helping those over-weight individuals return to a more desirable size.

But just as a weight gain or loss is gradual, so also should a change-over to more natural foods be gradual. A housewife intent on losing twenty pounds by using a natural foods diet should not plan an overnight revolution in the kitchen, otherwise she may well wind up with a revolution among her family! So bring the benefits of natural foods to your table slowly, and just as excess pounds will disappear, so also will non-dieters be weaned to the natural dishes you prepare. Not only the improvement in taste, particularly in green vegetables, but the exciting additions to various dishes will soon overcome any complaints over the disappearance of certain food items. Cooking naturally can also help forestall any weight problems in the future, for as we have said before, the right amounts of the right foods result in the body settling down to the right weight.

Chapter Three

Planning A Balanced Natural Food Menu

Before we get down to specific diets for those
with a weight problem, we want to detail the basic
essentials of menu preparation using natural
foods.

Many people are not aware of the basic food
groups that should be included in daily meals to
insure adequate nutrition. There are four basic
groups: protein; fruit and vegetables; milk and
milk products; grain products. Everyone should
include the right proportion of each of these
groups in the daily diet to make sure the body
receives all the elements necessary for proper
tissue maintenance and health.

Nutritionists generally recommend two servings
daily of protein. This can be in the form of meat,
poultry, fish, eggs or cheese. As we saw earlier,
the minimum meat requirement is only three

ounces, so anyone who has eggs and bacon for breakfast, plus a serving of meat later, perhaps a hamburger for lunch or a meat dish for dinner, has more than fulfilled the daily protein requirement.

Four or more servings daily of fruit and vegetables are advised, one of which should be a citrus fruit that is a good source of Vitamin C.

Milk is recommended for all age groups: 3 to 4 glasses for growing children, 4 or more for teenagers, and 2 or more for adults; for those on a diet, stick to skim milk, naturally.

Four servings daily are suggested for grain products, i.e. bread and other items containing wheat or other grain. (For dieters: Remember the carbohydrates found in fruit, vegetables, milk, and grain products should not exceed 75 grams a day. See the following chapter.)

Remember that the quality and preparation of the food you eat has a bearing upon its nutritional value. A hamburger, for example, especially those cooked in restaurants, can be so overdone that much of the food value is destroyed. To alert you to the right selection of all four food groups, we will deal with them individually and stress how you can supplement the requirements with additional natural foods to increase the nutritional content of each meal.

For dieters, white fish is preferable to meat protein, as there is only 3 percent fat in white fish compared with 40 percent in most meats.

If you have a keen sense of smell, this will be helpful in selecting fish at the market, because fresh fish has a crisp, clean, fish odor. The older fish becomes, the more pungent is its smell. Any fish you buy fresh should be firm and not have any unpleasant odor. If you are buying whole fish, rather than fillets, the scales should be shiny and tight and the gills, slightly pink.

Cooking fish requires care, as the protein in fish will solidify over 150 degrees. Overcooked fish is milky, somewhat pulpy and crumbles almost like sawdust. Properly cooked, fish should be firm. To prevent losing the outer layer of fish in the cooking process, always roll the fish in wheat germ or bread crumbs before baking or frying. By frying we do not mean a skillet loaded with grease! You will do better to use lecithin to prevent sticking, place the pieces of fish in the pan, and cover with a lid, turning as soon as the bottom browns. Fish cooks rather quickly and requires close attention, not only to preserve food value, but also to enhance flavor and consistency. If desired, a little margarine may be used in cooking.

Buying frozen fish means you will lose out a little on flavor, and you will lose even more if you defrost by soaking the fish in a bowl of water. Instead, place the frozen package in the refrigerator (wrapped in saran to keep the odor in) until thawed. Then the pieces can be separated, patted dry with a paper towel and cooked. Defrosting in water means you end up with a pulpy mess, minus nutrients. There are many excellent fish recipes included later that provide a wide variety of dishes for various occasions.

The most common meat dishes in the country are steaks and hamburgers, but the good we experience from eating steak is often more psychological than physical, as liver by far surpasses steak in food value and essential nutrients. But many see little appeal in liver when compared to a charcoal broiled filet or porterhouse!

Which brings up the matter of cooking: The high heat inherent in charcoal broiling sears the outside of the cut, ostensibly to keep in the juices. True, but we end up with only the inside of the meat in truly acceptable condition. The outside is merely a useless crust. Far preferable is slow cooking—giving you *all* the meat tender, juicy and still with its original food value intact. Slow cooking also means you can purchase a cheaper grade of beef, thereby saving money and still getting your full quota of protein.

There are six official grades of beef in the United States: *U.S. Prime,* tender and juicy, because it comes from young cattle. The lean areas are well marbled, meaning many streaks of fat permeate the lean part, giving good flavor to the cut. *U.S. Choice,* which is tasty, but has less fat than prime. *U.S. Good,* still lower in fat content, but still with good flavor and acceptable tenderness. *U.S. Standard* comes from older cattle and requires more care in preparation to make it palatable. *U.S. Commercial* definitely needs long, slow cooking to bring out flavor and tenderness. Finally, there is *U.S. Utility,* the lowest and most inexpensive grade, usually lean and stringy, coming from older cows.

However, all six grades are government inspected and approved, and are equally nutritious. The difference is naturally in the cost, and if you want to cut down on meat prices (and who doesn't these days!) you can select one of the lower grades and take more time in preparation to bring out the best flavor and tenderness. There is nothing wrong with using the cheaper grades for stews, casseroles, meat loaf, hamburger and similar dishes.

For hamburger, you will do well to select a lower grade of beef and have your butcher grind it while you wait, cutting off all fat. You will end up with far better quality hamburger than the packaged type sold in plastic, which contains filler and fat that makes it a poor bargain, both in food value and for the money.

An excellent investment is a food grinder, which can be bought at most stores for around 30 dollars. With this, you can not only grind your own hamburger (also, fish for fish-burgers), but you can chop and slice raw vegetables for tempting salads and vegetable dishes. A food grinder also is a penny-saver; you can grind up leftover meats for casseroles and shepherd pies, adding flavorful natural products like grains, nuts and leftover vegetables to enhance flavor and nutritive value. A food blender is also a valuable kitchen appliance in relation to natural foods, enabling you to pulverize many different nuts and grain products to include in cooking various dishes. Even people who don't like nuts will often accept them when ground up and disguised in meat loaf, pies and stews.

Sandwich meats are an old stand-by for lunches, especially for the kids, and we recommend that you make your own rather than buy the packaged type, which contain a great deal of preservatives, chemicals and artificial color. Also, home-cooked and sliced cold cuts cost far less than the cellpohane-wrapped variety found in stores. And they are far higher in nutritive value—*natural* food value!

Fruit and vegetables usually come to us from the supermarket—and most of the items on the produce counters are acceptable. But if you can find a farmer and buy your greens fresh from the soil, you'll be that much ahead. An apple picked off the tree is far superior in food value to those picked weeks ago and kept fresh through refrigeration or chemical means. It is a general rule that *any* food deteriorates with age; the fresher fruit and vegetables are, the greater will be the food value you get from them. Road-side stalls are a good source of fresher produce than you get in large stores, as are some smaller groceries where you know the owner takes special care in purchasing his greens.

Watch particularly for bruises in fruit and scrapes and scratches on zucchini and similar items, because very often you will want to cook the vegetables whole, skin and all—the healthful, natural way. Many people are not aware that zucchini can be eaten raw, sliced thin and chopped in salads. Delicious!

In general, buy fruits and vegetables frequently and fresh. When you buy the frozen variety, stick to the basics (peas, beans, corn, carrots, broccoli, cauliflower, etc.) They may not be as rich in flavor and nutrients as strictly organically grown greens, but the difference is not that significant, particularly since pure organic vegetables usually are hard to find.

The secret to flavor *and* preserving vitamins and minerals is in the cooking. Too many people dump their vegetables into water and boil the goodness away. Far better for you to invest in a couple of stainless steel steamers that expand to fit any size pot. They sell in most stores for around three or four dollars and are well worth the investment. Placing a cupful of water in the pot, then the vegetables in the steamer above, and covering will give you crisp, tasty vegetables that you never dreamed possible. A good alternative to the steamer is using a regular double boiler. The vegetables go in the top without water. All fruit and vegetables contain at least 70 percent water, so they actually cook in their own juices, retaining all the natural goodness and flavor. Whichever way you prefer to cook, however, your vegetables should come off the burner while they are still slightly crisp. Their color will be better (especially green items like string beans and peas) and the taste, fantastic compared with the pulpy, over-cooked specimens usually served from a steam table in a restaurant.

Another tip for cooking *naturally:* Save any liquids from cooking vegetables (either the water or the liquid from steaming) and use it as a base for soups and stews. You will be utilizing the minerals and food value and adding natural flavor to your soup or stew. You can keep it refrigerated in a large pot or bottle until you have enough to brew up a batch of home-made soup.

While cooked vegetables have become a regular part of our daily menu, a natural food program suggests trying to utilize as many vegetables raw as you can. In fact, one serving daily of any vegetable should be in the form of a salad. (We have some salad tips in a later chapter.) No matter how careful you are in cooking, you do lose some food value; hence our recommendation for raw vegetables and salads. Raw fruit daily is also strongly advised: pure, natural orange juice for that all-important Vitamin C, plus an apple, peach or pear. If no fresh fruit is available, dried fruits are an excellent substitute. Canned fruit would be a last resort.

Certified raw milk is certainly better than the pasteurized. And milk products such as yogurt, buttermilk and cheese should be *natural* and not processed. For those concerned over weight, skim milk is recommended over whole milk, provided there is sufficient fat intake through other foods. Calcium needs fat to help it be absorbed into the body.

For those eager to put *on* weight, additional nutrition can be given to milk by stirring in a little powdered milk, which supplements the basic food value and makes a much richer tasting drink. For an even richer flavor and body, add a tablespoon of malt and a scoop of ice cream. This is a particularly good method of helping kids put on weight during their growing years, and it is certainly better for them than the malts served at most soda fountains.

In the final group, the grain products, we suggest no white bread at all, but strictly whole-wheat. Similarly, we suggest brown rice rather than white. The key to natural nutrition in the grain products is the word "unrefined", for in the refining process, much of the inherent goodness of the grain is either destroyed or removed. Most markets now carry whole-wheat bread, or stone-ground, but if for whatever reason, you prefer to stick to white bread, buy the kind that is made without chemical additives and preservatives.

In short, we recommend eliminating overly processed, packaged food items and substituting dishes that you make from scratch, using ingredients that you know are pure and uncontaminated with chemical additives, preservatives and emulsifiers, none of which do the body metabolism any good. This does not mean throwing away your accustomed recipes and established ideas on menu preparation; it merely means modifying them and using different ingredients.

For example, many cooks use commercial bouillon, either the powdered type or the canned liquid, as a base for soups, stews or just for a refreshing change from tea or coffee. By making your own, you will not only save money, but avoid the chemical additives in the commercial product. How? Simple as ABC: A) Add water to a large pot; B) Add beef bones and beef scraps; C) Cook slowly at a gentle simmer with whatever natural herbs you prefer, plus onion, garlic, and a touch of your favorite sauce (Worcestershire, Tabasco, etc.). The longer you simmer, the richer and more flavorful will be your bouillon, which you can keep refrigerated or frozen. For chicken flavor, use chicken bones and scraps instead of beef. Both are excellent bases in which to cook your rice, giving it taste and added food value.

Bread crumbs are often used in preparing various dishes. Switch to wheat germ, or softened soy grits, both valuable sources of natural nourishment.

For those recipes in which you presently use white enriched flour, change to unbleached white flour, or coarsely ground whole wheat flour, or Cornell mix which is a formula developed by Cornell University for extra-rich bread: Place in a measuring cup one tablespoon each of soy flour and non-fat dry milk powder, and one teaspoon of wheat germ; then fill the cup with unbleached flour. You can mix this yourself, or buy it prepackaged; the mixture works in any recipe in place of regular white flour, but provides far more natural nourishment.

In baking bread or pastries, replace each cup of white flour with ¾ cup of whole wheat flour and ¼ cup of wheat germ. For cakes, cookies or other sweet baked goods, replace a cup of white flour with ½ cup of whole wheat pastry flour and ½ cup of rice flour.

For items such as waffles or pancakes, use half unbleached flour and half whole wheat flour. The following can also be used in place of white flour: arrowroot flour, barley flour, cornstarch, buckwheat flour, coarse cornmeal, oat flour, soy flour, rice flour, or any other of the grain flours you may like to try. Quantities are usually less than for white flour, and experimentation will help you determine which one appeals most to you from a flavor standpoint.

We are all so used to certain tastes in baked goods that switching to natural grain products has, of necessity, to be a trial and error matter as everyone has their particular taste preference; some are a little more distinctive than others, but all contribute greater nutritional value than white flour and should therefore be tested before you arrive at a final choice.

Instead of white flour for thickening gravies and stews, try arrowroot, potato or tapioca flour, which can also be used for custards and souffles.

To replace refined granulated sugar, you can use honey, ¾ cup equalling 1 cup of sugar. If the recipe contains liquid, reduce this by ¼ cup when using honey; if dry, add 4 tablespoons of flour to compensate for the liquid in the honey. A cup of sugar can also be replaced by a cup of sorghum syrup, or 1¼ to 1½ cups of maple, carob or malt syrups. Remember that natural sweeteners are more potent than white sugar and also have a slightly different taste which many people prefer to sugar.

For extra flavor, use sea salt in place of table salt; also vegetable salt or ground kelp, which contribute additional mineral content to your menu.

We mentioned brewer's yeast before, but we stress again that you should add this sparingly to any recipe, such as for soups or stews or pies, as it has a distinctive taste. Experimentation is your only guide in using brewer's yeast in your various dishes, but it cannot be recommended too highly as a natural source of vitamins and minerals.

Turning to nature will eliminate many of the dietary problems that can arise from indiscreet consumption of those foods which modern ingenuity has provided. As we said, many of these are highly tempting, taste good and please the palate—but are not always good for one, especially in the area of weight control. Many people believe that "going natural" involves some sort of tedious self-discipline that takes all the joy out of eating. Far from it! For most cooks, switching to natural ingredients has been the start of intriguing explorations in the kitchen. The experimental phase of cooking naturally increases our knowledge of the various items, how they work, and what they do; above all, as time passes, you'll see what they do for family health, with increased energy, vitality and general good health for every member of the household.

So if you're going to fight those extra pounds, switch to natural foods *now!* Even without a weight problem, you'll benefit from improved general health, and a natural balance of protein, fats and carbohydrates, vitamins and minerals in your daily food intake. For remember: It is the *balance* of all the essential foods that counts.

Chapter Four

Getting Down To Dieting

We are trained from infancy to be over-weight. How many times have you seen women gathered around a new-born infant, gurgling with delight and making comments over the chubbiness of the child? A less plump baby usually elicits a sympathetic remark about the "poor skinny thing"—showing how we equate heaviness with health, at least in babies!

Nothing could be further from the truth; a growing infant has enough problems without uncomfortable rolls of flesh that interfere with general mobility and which can often cause unpleasant skin rashes. Many far-thinking doctors are now advising mothers to put their babies on skim milk at nine months to cut down on calories and help establish a pattern of *not* over-eating.

Many of our eating habits are predicated on the conditioned oral response, which stems from childhood. A baby nurses at its mother's breast or the bottle. Between feedings a pacifier is popped into the mouth to hopefully stop the cries of the child. The mouth becomes the focal point for satisfaction, reflected in later life with constant snacking to allay feelings of frustration. After puberty, the oral response is replaced in part by sexual desires, but when these are thwarted, an individual turns or reverts to oral gratification. Sexually dissatisfied men and women often find a substitute pleasure in eating, with the unhappy result of overweight.

Which brings us to a pertinent question: What causes an overweight condition? From a physical standpoint, it is usually eating too much or eating the wrong foods. But, basically, shoveling food into the stomach is the beginning of all our problems regarding body weight.

Eating is essential for the sustenance of the body, for maintenance and replacement of tissue and the creation of energy for our daily activities. Primitive man ate when he was hungry and his diet consisted mainly of animal flesh or protein.

Modern man has increased his intake of food to include a variety of items that have less to do with nutrition than with sensual satisfaction. Eating has become a social function, a pleasant interlude in the daily routine. The suburban housewife's morning coffee-klatsch or the English habit of four o'clock tea has little to do with the actual need for sustenance; rather these occasions offer the opportunity to socialize, to combine chatter with calories that do little but fill the stomach and expand the waistline. Even regular meals have items which are used as sensual gratification rather than nutritional need; for example, rich desserts. Many children eat their meat and vegetables only as a means of being given those sought-after sweets that follow. "No dessert if you don't finish your beans," threatens the mother, wondering why her children don't attack the main course with enthusiasm. How can they, when they have been programmed since birth to reach for the candy?

Among existing primitive tribes in Africa and the South Seas, the traditional Western menu format is unknown; dessert, if any, is fresh fruit. The result: Only rarely does one see an overweight man or woman in these areas. They are *naturally* well-proportioned. If we still walked or ran instead of using the automobile and if we had a less exotic diet, our weight problems would be almost non-existent!

Modern man hopefully has the intelligence to realize the reason behind his problems, and for those who seriously want to get back in shape, this book can point the way. But, remember, once you are aware of the ground rules, it is up to you to play the game!

To get back to your natural shape, you must be aware of what your natural shape is. The human anatomy has been divided into three basic types:

(1) The *ectomorph*, who is tall and slender, resembling the test tube in shape.

(2) The *endomorph*, who is stocky and thick set, sometimes called the "barrel" type.

(3) The *mesomorph*, who is the traditional athletic type, with broad shoulders and narrow waist, and muscular conformation; sometimes called the "wine-glass" type.

No amount of exercise or dieting will change

your physical type, so you will do well to remember the old maxim: "God grant me the serenity to accept the things I cannot change; courage to change the things I can; and wisdom to know the difference."

But whatever type you are, an overweight condition *is* something you can change, and hopefully you will have the courage to stick to a new regimen in your eating habits that will bring about the desired change, and be wise enough to maintain it afterwards. While you may still have to restrict your food intake to preserve your desired proportions, eating natural foods will minimize the possibility of a recurring weight problem, as well as improving your general health and well-being.

An overweight ectomorph usually shows the excess around the waist, which is the first area in the body to respond to over-eating. Normally tall and slender, your arms and legs might remain slender, but there's that objectionable bulge at the midriff.

The endomorph simply blows up like a balloon, becoming fat and flabby all over.

The mesomorph, who is the least susceptible to weight problems, shows excess weight around the middle, together with a layer of flab over the normally firm, tight muscles with which he is blessed.

No amount of dieting or exercise will turn a "barrel" into a "wine-glass" or a "test-tube"— but getting down to a natural weight level will result in a healthy body and an acceptable shape.

The same diet does not necessarily apply to all three types or even all persons of the same type. Occupations and life-styles must be considered, too. A badly overweight endomorph may be engaged in heavy construction work. We have seen thick-set laborers working on building sites, the size of their stomachs attesting to their daily drop-in at the tavern! An endomorph, therefore, could not survive on 900 calories a day, due to the nature of his work. But 1500 to 2000 calories a day, plus limiting carbohydrates to 50-75 grams daily, would help him reduce, and is certainly an improvement over 5000 calories a day, which is what many large, heavy-set men consume.

Our diet formulas, therefore, are divided into groups to match not only basic physical type, but also nature of occupation. A woman working on her feet in a department store all day will need more calories than the office secretary seated behind the desk. In our breakdown, we give broad categories which are flexible, and it will be up to you to assess your needs after studying your particular situation, taking into account your basic type and your occupation.

The following will help you understand the reasoning behind more than mere caloric limitation: For some people, a mere limiting of calories may work fine, but with the majority, more is involved, stemming from the intake of carbohydrates which, as glucose, are the building blocks of the fatty tissue in the body. In reducing, we want to conserve the muscle protein mass and break down the fatty tissue. Nutritionists have also found that the taking of polyunsaturated fats, such as corn oil, in the absence of glucose (carbohydrates), helps eliminate fat. So, basically, your protein intake, plus 2-3 ounces daily of polyunsaturated fats, and restricting your carbohydrates to 50-75 grams, adds up to maintenance of muscle protein mass while fatty tissue is broken down. Remember that on any type of diet, the aim is to conserve the muscle protein mass at the same time as fat is removed so that we end up with a healthy, normal body weight with all the tissues in good shape, and none of that "haggard, starved" look.

Your own understanding of the principles of nutrition, plus cultivating the necessary self-discipline and also the right positive outlook, will insure success. Switching to more natural food items in your daily menu is *not* a tedious chore. We have already shown that eating naturally is just what the name implies, and a positive approach to the many new food items for your kitchen will aid you in establishing a natural routine to replace the one that has obviously led to your weight problem. Following a natural food diet is no gimmick or magic formula; it merely means eating the way we are *supposed* to.

Our minds have to work *with* our bodies. So make your decision and stick to it; and be happy about the new lease on life that natural foods most assuredly will provide—along with better health, more energy and brighter spirits. Both food and exercise have an effect upon our mental responses and our mental health.

One immediate reaction to going on any kind of a diet is: "I'm going to feel hungry all the time!" Not so with a natural food diet as outlined here, for again we are breaking with tradition. We have been programmed to presume that three meals a day is the required routine. But in any attempt at weight loss, it is not the number of times you eat that counts, but the amount of calories you consume.

As 1000 calories mean less bulk than 5000, it *is* possible that a dieter will feel pangs of hunger with only three meals a day. But we give you the alternative in the natural foods diet: You can have *six* meals a day, instead of three, if you prefer. In fact, from experience with many patients, it is clear that the six-times-a-day routine works very well, with no hunger pangs, and little of the trauma usually associated with losing weight.

Your immediate question is probably: "How can six portions of food possibly help one *lose* weight? The answer is: The daily caloric intake is divided up between the six meals so that one does not over-eat, but still there is something in the stomach to make you feel satisfied.

Naturally, the six meals are not full-course dinners, but then anyone going on a diet has no business eating a full course meal anyway! But the extra three eating periods do keep away the hunger pangs and do not provide excess calories, as allowed, but the determining factor is the amount most between-meal snacks do.

With some patients, only three meals a day are of over-weight and the degree of weight loss expected. Common-sense would indicate that a heavy-set laborer who is fifty pounds overweight would not achieve the best results on the six-meal-a-day routine; but the office worker who wants to trim off fifteen pounds could very well find six-meals-a-day a preferable method to three-meals-a-day.

As we have stressed before, the psychological aspects are most important in weight control and dieting. Many people find their courage waning after the first few days if the hunger pangs prove too traumatic. The result: Many give up before the battle is won! So that empty feeling is a signal that you should switch to six meals a day.

If one limits carbohydrates to 50-75 grams a day, what are the maximum calories allowable? As a general rule, to reduce weight, a rough daily average of 1600 calories is prescribed. However, some patients will be limited to 800, while others need more. Daily work load and bodily type are keys to assessing the needed caloric intake.

How does one determine the right amount? Check the following chart, dividing occupations into three types: light, medium and heavy work.

Light work would include sedentary positions (clerks, typists, writers, artists, most desk jobs). Medium work would be that which includes a certain amount of footwork (department store employees, doctors' and dentists' assistants and nurses, salesmen, housewives, professional people who walk a lot). Heavy work includes mostly manual labor (construction workers, mechanics, builders, carpenters, etc.).

In each of the three divisions, there are three further breakdowns determined by the amount of weight loss desired: slight, average or maximum. A slight weight loss could be from five to fifteen pounds. Average would be fifteen to twenty-five pounds. Maximum would be anything over twenty-five pounds. So our chart reads as follows:

EMPLOYMENT:	LIGHT WORK (1)	MEDIUM WORK (2)	HEAVY WORK (3)
DESIRED WEIGHT LOSS:	Slight (3)	Slight (3)	Slight (3)
	Average (2)	Average (2)	Average (2)
	Maximum (1)	Maximum (1)	Maximum (1)

To work out your maximum caloric intake, take the number from the top line (type of work) and add it to the number opposite the desired weight loss, then multiply by 400, which will give you your maximum number of calories daily.

Example: An office worker wants to lose 15 pounds. Light work (1) plus an average weight loss (2) equals (3). Multiply by 400, making 1200, which would be the maximum calories to be consumed daily.

Example: A construction worker wants to lose thirty pounds. Heavy work (3) plus a maximum weight loss (1) equals (4). Multiply this by 400 gives 1600 calories, the maximum number advisable.

Using this table, no one can come up with less than 800 calories a day, or more than 2400, with the average being from 1200 to 1600 calories, an acceptable level for weight loss without sacrificing essential basic nutrition. Don't forget the 50-75 grams of carbohydrates applies, no matter what the calorie limit is, together with 3 servings of protein daily, and 2-3 ounces of polyunsaturated fats.

The only exception to this chart would be for individuals engaged in extremely heavy work that places a great physical burden on them, in which case the caloric intake can be upped to 2000, but never more.

There are many theories regarding frequency of meals while on a diet. Some doctors recommend a hearty breakfast, little if any lunch, and a good meal at night. Others lean towards almost nothing for breakfast, a light lunch and a large meal at night. Each individual has his particular preference to which he has become accustomed over the years, but without exception, it is far healthier and better for your body to eat more often, and smaller quantities, than the old idea of starving all day and filling up at night, which places a strain on the metabolic processes, and leads to a lack of balance in the body mechanism.

Not only must the *balance* of *foods* be correct, but also the *balance* of *intake:* Six small amounts daily are infinitely preferable to one or two larger meals. Small amounts keep the stomach happy and the mind at rest, while the restriction of quantity brings about the desired weight loss. The use of natural foods increases the pure food elements inherent in the daily intake of sustenance and helps avoid filling up with bulk that has questionable nutritional value.

An example of a good balanced daily menu with less than 1200 calories and approximately 75 grams of carbohydrates could be the following:

Meal	Calories	Carbo-hydrates (GRAMS)
BREAKFAST:		
One poached or boiled egg	80	.4
One slice whole wheat bread	55	11.9
Margarine for bread (or toast)	25	—
½ cup tomato juice	23	5.2
Black coffee, tea or Sanka	0	0
MID-MORNING SNACK:		
One medium fresh peach	38	9.6
LUNCH:		
One cup cottage cheese (or cheese snacks)	200	6.2
One fresh plum	25	6.9

	Calories	Carbo- hydrates (GRAMS)
Small lettuce and tomato salad	45	7.0
Low-cal mayonnaise	24	.1
MID-AFTERNOON SNACK:		
½ cup yogurt	76	6.0
DINNER:		
One slice roast beef	270	—
Serving cooked green beans	16	3.3
” ” carrots	25	5.8
½ cup cubed cantaloupe	24	6.1
Black coffee, tea or Sanka	0	0
MID-EVENING SNACK:		
Cheese and apple slices	100	2.0
Total Calories and Carbohydrates	1026	70.3

NOTE: No alcohol, but if you must, don't forget to
count the calories!

Naturally, there is almost a limitless variety of
dishes from which to put together a diet that
will appeal to your particular taste, yet not exceed the prescribed caloric count you determine
for your particular situation.

In working out your diet, don't forget the four
basic food groups: protein, fruit and vegetables,
milk and milk products, grains. Even a reducing
diet must be balanced, just as a normal diet should
contain the right proportion of all food groups to
insure the body getting all its essential nutrition.

In the ensuing chapters, we include recipes and
hints on food preparation that will enable you to
expand your present selection of dishes, but never

at the cost of calories. All the dishes we list are rich in nutrients but low in calories. Prepared with natural ingredients, these dishes will prove tempting items on your table, considering your appetite and taste at the same time as they help control your weight.

Chapter Five

Healthful Breakfasts

There are many hints that help cut down unwanted and unnecessary calories that creep into the cooking of all meals, particularly breakfasts, which often involve frying—fried eggs, fried bacon, and so on. We won't deny that a good hot breakfast is preferred by many people, especially during the colder months. A low-calorie cold cereal is not always the most appealing way to start the day when the snow is inches deep outside!

We'll start out with the most popular standby: eggs. As most dieters will stick with one egg, there is a way to make a single egg appear more than it is. Separate the yolk and, using a high speed electric mixer, beat the white in a wide bowl, adding a tablespoon of cold water. Continue beating until the whites are fluffy and very firm and dry. Now add the yolk, together with salt to taste, or your favorite herbs or a drop of sauce. Continue beating until blended. The mixture will be thick and rich looking. Add sea salt to taste.

Pour into a skillet with a rounded bottom (better known as an omelet pan) that has been wiped with lecithin or vegetable oil. Peanut oil is excellent for this. You will probably need a rubber spatula to scrape the beaten egg from the bowl. The skillet should be fairly hot, so that the egg sizzles when it is poured in. Cover with a lid, turn the heat down and cook until the bottom is lightly browned (about a minute to a minute-and-a-half). Using a nylon spatula, ease the egg over (it is too light to be flipped) and cook until browned. Then slide off and serve. Unless eaten right away, the one-egg omelet will deflate, but still be tasty and appear much larger than one egg poached, boiled or fried. Psychologically, this helps with the essential feeling of "having had enough"!

Cooking eggs as they come from the shell should also be done in a rounded skillet, using lecithin to cut down on the calories inherent in butter or oil. For those who crave more flavor, about half a teaspoon of margarine may be added, but no more. Don't forget to count the amount you use in cooking when adding up your calories!

If your diet allows two eggs, you can make an interesting dish as follows: Separate the eggs and beat the whites until stiff, using two tablespoons of chicken broth (hopefully your own home-made, as described earlier!). If desired, you may use water and a teaspoon of dehydrated chicken bouillon; but the home-made is preferable from a natural food standpoint. Add the yolks, beat until blended and cook slowly as detailed above for one egg. This two-egg omelet dish, if cooked with one teaspoon of butter in the skillet, adds up to only 190 calories.

For those who like eggs "over-easy" but don't want the fat usually necessary to cook them this way, here's a tip: Place the eggs in a skillet that has been wiped with either lecithin or oil. Cover with a lid. After about a minute, by which time the bottom should be firm, gently add a tablespoon of water without lifting the lid. Merely let the water in under the edge of the lid, then replace it at once, turning the heat up. The water naturally steams and cooks the top of the eggs, giving them the same appearance as "over-easy", but with hardly any grease. If you prefer your eggs "over-hard", just leave them in a while longer.

Oven-baked eggs provide additional opportunities for tasty breakfast dishes that are low in calories. A baked cheese omelet is particularly tempting and easy to make. For each serving required, mix the following ingredients: two egg whites (beaten until stiff), one egg yolk, ¼ teaspoon sea salt, ¼ cup solid low-fat cottage cheese, two teaspoons vegetable oil. Place in a shallow dish that has been wiped with lecithin or oil, and bake for 20 minutes at 400 degrees, or until omelet is brown on top. Each serving contains 190 calories.

For those with a sweet tooth, this same baked omelet can be varied by adding ¼ cup crushed fruit, such as pineapple, apple, peach or orange, over the top just before serving.

For those who like a tang, such as you get with Spanish foods, here's a spicy omelet that won't upset your calorie count: Place two eggs in a blender, then add one small tomato, a teaspoon of minced fresh onion, ¼ teaspoon sea salt, ¼ teaspoon black pepper, a pinch of garlic salt, a pinch of cayenne, and a few drops of Tabasco sauce. Blend at low speed for 3 seconds. The mixture can either be cooked in a skillet or baked in the oven as described above, until the top is brown. Each serving contains only 190 calories.

From Spain to India: How about curried eggs? These provide a different and unusual variation to the breakfast menu. Use the same recipe and cooking method as the preceding, but substitute a tablespoon of beef bouillon for the tomato, and add ¼ teaspoon curry powder. For a particularly hot dish, you may increase 'the curry powder, but be careful! This curry omelet forms an appealing main dish for a brunch, together with a tossed salad garnished with almonds and sliced banana.

Any of the above omelet recipes can be varied in the cooking by pouring the mixture into poaching cups and poaching instead of baking or frying. Be sure not to fill the cups more than half-full, because the mixture puffs up as it cooks.

Natural food toppings add a nutritious and flavorful extra touch to any egg dish: a mixture of equal amounts of sunflower seeds, sesame seeds and flaxseed, raw nuts and fresh coconut. Grind these in a blender into rough granules and sprinkle over the cooked eggs. This addition is especially tasty with a Spanish omelet or curried eggs.

Lovers of Chinese food will enjoy a sprout omelet, which is even lower in calories than the above. For each serving, combine 1½ tablespoons minced celery; 1½ tablespoons minced green pepper; 1½ tablespoons sprouts (bean sprouts are the best for this dish); 1½ tablespoons chopped fresh onion (Bermuda or green onions); ¼ cup chicken bouillon. Simmer gently in a small pan for about two minutes. While this mixture is cooking, pour one egg, well-beaten, into a skillet and cover. Cook until the bottom is browned and the top fairly firm. Slide onto a plate and cover with the cooked sprout mixture, sprinkling lightly with soy sauce for extra seasoning. Only 125 calories per serving! If you intend serving this dish to four or more persons, bake the eggs in the oven and add the vegetable mixture a few minutes before serving. Place on the table with a final garnishing of chopped parsley.

Maybe this would be a good time to mention that food often tastes better when it looks appetizing (that psychological factor again), so don't neglect those final garnishing touches. If you have several different colored serving platters, choose one that will complement the color of the food: a contrast or a similar shade, plus shredded lettuce or parsley around the edges. Even a sprinkling of paprika over white or yellow foods (potatoes, rice, eggs) can add appetite interest.

Let's move on to another item that is always popular, but which many dieters feel beyond their caloric limit: pancakes. We'd like to stress that while pancakes *can* be hazardous for those watching their weight, we've prepared several recipes that are well within the bounds of a low-calorie diet.

First, some tips on preparation and cooking: Never add fat or oil to the recipe for pancakes, for obvious reasons, and don't use it for frying the pancakes, either. A non-stick surface electric griddle is best: The temperature is controllable, and 400-425 degrees is about right for any type of batter. As an added precaution, you can wipe the surface with lecithin, which would also be advisable if you use a regular skillet instead of a griddle. Without a temperature guide, use the old-fashioned but still reliable test of a drop of water. When a drop bounces over the hot skillet, begin cooking.

Finally, a psychological ploy: Never make your pancakes too large. Not only are pancakes difficult to handle and turn, but two large ones never seem as much as four small ones, even though the actual batter content may be the same.

Should you prefer to buy a packaged pancake mix, buy the buckwheat or soy flour mixes: only 90 calories per ounce, with 10 percent protein for buckwheat and 14 percent for soy. You can also add bulk, flavor and very few extra calories by including finely chopped fresh fruit with the pancake batter. Apple, pineapple or blueberries are especially delicious cooked in pancakes. Here is a recipe that includes blueberries and each 3-4" pancake contains only 30 calories.

Mix together (by hand or slow-speed electric mixer): 1 egg, 1 cup skim milk, 3 teaspoons honey, ½ teaspoon sea salt, 2 teaspoons baking powder, 1 cup whole wheat, buckwheat or soy flour, ½ cup unsweetened blueberries. Add the fruit last, after the other ingredients have been thoroughly blended. Make sure your griddle or skillet is hot enough, then drop the batter on to make pancakes 3-4" across. Cook until the bubbles have stopped rising, the top is barely dry, and the bottom nicely browned. Turn and brown, then serve.

If you have an electric griddle, you can add to the fun and tastiness of pancakes by placing the griddle on the table and cooking pancakes to order, rather than cooking up a lot in advance and having to keep them in the oven. There's nothing more tempting than a freshly cooked pancake, hot off the griddle, steaming with natural fresh flavor and goodness!

Plain pancakes can be made as follows: 1¼ cups whole wheat, buckwheat or soy flour; 2½ teaspoons baking powder; ½ teaspoon sea salt; 1 egg; 1¼ cups skim milk. Mix by hand or with an electric mixer. Some cooks insist that pancake batter should be lumpy, but we find that the smoother the batter, the better the consistency of the pancake, hence the value of an electric mixer to handle the blending chore.

Cook as described above. Each 3-4" pancake contains only 35 calories.

An electric blender will enable you to make low-calorie cottage cheese pancakes that are really delicious. Blend the following first, at medium speed until creamy: 2 eggs; 1 cup low-fat cottage cheese; ¾ cup skim milk. Now add: 1 cup whole wheat, buckwheat or soy flour; ½ teaspoon sea salt; ½ teaspoon baking soda. Continue blending until creamy. You will possibly have to scrape the mixture down from the sides to make sure everything is blended together thoroughly. Cook as described before. This recipe, like all pancake recipes, can have unsweetened fresh fruit added if desired—just the fruit, not any juice (which will make the mixture too thin and watery to rise properly).

Regarding the use of various flours, we suggest you experiment (perhaps half whole wheat, half soy; or varying proportions) to arrive at a mixture that pleases your palate the most. Some very tempting pancakes can be made by mixing different flours to give a different taste, as each flour has its particular characteristic.

Yogurt pancakes are very nutritious and rich in protein. Combine 8 ounces of plain yogurt, either in a blender or mixing bowl, with 1¼ cups of the flour of your choice; ½ teaspoon sea salt; 1 teaspoon baking soda; a pinch of baking powder; 1 egg yolk; ¼ cup skim milk; 2 egg whites. Mix until smooth and creamy, then cook as before. Yogurt pancakes are especially good with chopped apple, or a tablespoon of apple sauce added before cooking, and a little cinnamon sprinkled over each pancake.

For a special treat, you can try German pancakes, which in reality are more a souffle than a pancake, being cooked in one large skillet (ovenproof) rather than as individual pancakes, and individual servings are cut from the finished dish.

Blend together: 1 cup flour (half whole wheat, half soy is very good for this recipe); 1 cup skim milk; 5 eggs; ½ teaspoon baking powder; ½ teaspoon sea salt. Use an electric mixer or a blender until the ingredients are smooth and creamy.

Use a large (9-10") skillet, making sure the handle will survive oven temperatures, or better still, a ceramic-type casserole that is not too deep. Cover the inside with lecithin or wipe with about a tablespoon of vegetable oil. Pour in the entire batter mixture and cook over medium heat for 1-1½ minutes, or until the bottom is set. Then place in a hot oven (425 degrees) for approximately 20 minutes, or until the mixture is browned nicely and fluffed up.

Serve at once at the table, filling the middle with chopped fresh fruit or a mixture of fruit and yogurt. You should get about six good servings from this recipe, each serving being around 200 calories, which includes about a tablespoon of fruit, such as peaches, pears or apples.

From German to Jewish: Have you ever tried blintzes for breakfast? Many people like blintzes as a late evening snack, but they make a great breakfast dish. There are actually two types: the plain, very thin pancake, made about 6-7" across, using the regular pancake recipe given earlier, into which you place a tablespoon of sour cream, then roll up the pancake and top it with preserves or fresh, crushed fruit of your choice. Strawberries are particularly good as a blintz topping. A blintz made in this manner averages out to about 50-60 calories.

The second type uses cottage cheese as the main base for the filling, and the blintzes are baked in the oven, after cooking one side only on the pan or griddle. The cottage cheese filling is made as follows: Blend together ¾ cup cottage cheese; 1 teaspoon honey; ½ teaspoon vanilla; ½ teaspoon cinnamon (optional); 1 egg white; pinch of sea salt. Roll your half-cooked pancake with about a tablespoon of this filling and bake in a moderate oven (350 degrees) for fifteen minutes. Each blintz gives about 50-55 calories. The oven-baked blintzes are a little dryer than those with sour cream filling; try them both to determine your preference. They're both good!

Syrups for pancakes can be made from natural ingredients and give you almost an infinite variety of toppings to use, all low in calories. Merely simmer together finely chopped fresh fruit with honey (1 cup fruit to ¾ cup honey), then add sufficient water to make it a suitable consistency for pouring; or if you prefer, use it thick. The thickness naturally depends on the length of time you simmer the mixture. Peaches, apricots, raspberries and blueberries make excellent syrups for pancakes. And for a real zingy taste, have you tried tomatoes? Be sure and remove the skins in boiling water, then liquefy the tomatoes in a blender before starting the simmering. Delicious!

Some of these syrups, when cool, can also be used over ice cream. A tablespoon is more than enough to use per serving, because of sweetness and calories.

A variation on pancakes is French toast, which works out to about 85 calories per slice—a little rich, but if you can afford the calories, why not? Use whole wheat or high protein bread slices, dipped in the following mixture: 2 large eggs; ½ teaspoon sea salt; ½ teaspoon vanilla; ¾ cup skim milk. The bread slices should be dipped and soaked in the mixture, then cooked in a skillet or on a griddle the same way as you would pancakes, turning after the bottom browns nicely.

French toast can also be topped with fresh fruit and cottage cheese, which would bring the calorie count per slice up to around 250 calories, but a filling and nutritious, tasty breakfast.

Many people do not consider a breakfast a meal unless a meat is included, traditionally bacon or sausage. Sadly, both these pork products are more than 50 percent fat, which makes them rather unappealing from a caloric standpoint.

However, bacon and sausages can be treated to reduce the fat content. Instead of frying bacon, place the strips on a narrow mesh rack over a tray and place in a 450 degree oven. The fat drains off, leaving the bacon crisp and vastly reduced in calories. A very crisp slice of bacon contains between 40-50 calories. The crisper it is, the less fat and the fewer calories. Canadian bacon is even better: one slice, broiled, contains approximately 16 calories. Another alternative for the bacon-fiend is to buy a lean, cooked ham (only 70 calories per ounce!) and cut bacon-strip pieces off and heat in the oven; never fry. Even less caloric is smoked chicken or smoked turkey, with about 38 calories per ounce, which can also be served as a breakfast meat for a change; cut a slice and warm it in the oven like the cooked ham.

Sausage can be easily de-fatted by pricking the links with a sharp fork and dropping them into a pot of boiling water and letting them steep for five to ten minutes with the flame turned down. This melts the fat, after which the sausages can be baked or broiled as usual, but not fried.

An even better way to satisfy the sausage hunger without pork is to make your own beef sausage patties. A pound of lean round steak, finely ground, and mixed with 1 teaspoon of poultry seasoning, ½ teaspoon garlic salt and pepper to taste will give you about 8 patties with only about 75 calories apiece.

Similarly, you can buy beef bacon which contains only 115 calories per ounce against 190 in pork bacon. Beef bacon runs a little more than pork, but you get more meat because of the lower fat content.

If you have your own meat grinder, you can add another meat variation to your breakfast menu by grinding up small pieces of beef leftovers (or ham), running it through several times until you end up with a paste, similar to the cans of deviled ham obtainable in the market. Adding a tablespoon of this to an egg and mixing in a blender will give you the base for a tasty omelet that puts the nourishment of eggs and meat together in the same dish.

We are going to close our breakfast chapter on a nostalgic note: How many of you remember an old Betty Grable movie in which she fixed breakfast for Dick Haymes with a dish that, for a while, became known as "Betty Grable eggs"? Using a slice of whole-wheat bread or high-protein bread, you can use the same recipe for a low-calorie, nutritious dish. There's really very little to it, but it has great eye-appeal: Merely take a slice of bread and cut or pull out a circle in the middle about two inches across.

Drop the bread on a heated skillet (wiped with oil or lecithin) and top with one egg, allowing the yolk to settle in the cut-out circle, and the white to flow evenly over the rest of the slice. Cover with a deep lid and allow to cook until the egg is firm. The bread beneath will be browned (toasted). About 130 calories of great natural taste!

Depending upon the daily calories you have

worked out for yourself, you should allow yourself a respectable quantity for breakfast. Remember that the body has been without food for eight hours and, although during sleep there is no strenuous physical activity to use up energy, the basic metabolism still continues, so that on arising, most people will benefit from a good breakfast. And one can have a good breakfast and still keep the calorie count to 200-300.

We suggest you make a list of all the various recipes and food items you want to include in your breakfast menu, together with the appropriate calorie count. Include prepared dishes as well as basic food products. Then make a weekly schedule, perhaps staggering eggs to three times a week, pancakes twice, and so on, until you get a well-balanced variety that includes all the essential food groups as well as maintaining your desired caloric limit.

If you decide on the six-meals-a-day routine, you can easily cut some calories out of breakfast and add them to your mid-morning snack; perhaps only an egg for breakfast, but whole wheat toast and coffee a few hours later. The main determining factor will be your total daily calories, worked out from the chart in the preceding chapter. If you only wish to lose a few pounds, you can be a little more lenient with yourself than someone who plans to lose fifty pounds!

But whatever your goal, don't think you're doing yourself any good by settling for black coffee and cigarettes. Neither are to be highly recommended as being beneficial for one's health. In fact, while we're on the subject of coffee, we suggest you limit your daily intake while you're on a diet, for reasons of your nerves. Coffee, containing caffeine, is a stimulant—and, in actuality, an *artificial* stimulant that places a strain on the nervous system as well as being an irritant for people with heart problems and gastric complaints.

Cutting down on your calories means you're going to be under a psychological strain, whether you feel it or not, so any unnatural stimulation doesn't help any. Far better for you to choose fresh fruit juice instead, which will also lessen the desire for cigarettes. It's a well-known fact that smokers automatically reach for a cigarette with coffee; the two tastes seem to go together.

So remember what breakfast means: *breaking* the *fast*. As such, this means food, not coffee and cigarettes! If you can, switch to a decaffeinated coffee not only during your diet, but permanently. There are many brands out now which equal regular coffee in flavor—and eliminating that caffeine from your system will have a marked effect on your outlook and peace of mind. Too often, nervousness can be traced to too much coffee in the diet. If, by reason of taste preference, you do not enjoy a decaffeinated coffee, drink tea as an alternative, which is far less stimulating than coffee. The traditional British calm has sometimes been said to result from the English habit of tea-drinking in preference to coffee.

From a natural food standpoint, you will do best to minimize tea and coffee in your daily intake of liquids, especially coffee. And as we've said before, no alcohol, though if this is asking too much, make sure you count the calories, even for a glass of wine!

As fruit juices seem to be standard breakfast fare, along with bacon and eggs, we want to remind you that orange juice has 110 calories per cup. Tomato juice, only 45. While orange juice is a good source of Vitamin C, there are other equally good sources to draw on, and putting tomato juice on your breakfast menu will save you those extra 60 calories. Tomato juice is also good to put down for your mid-morning snack.

A final thought: On cold winter mornings, many people enjoy a bowl of hot cereal, such as oatmeal, which contains only 130 calories. Complete with honey and skim milk, this can provide a nourishing and filling breakfast. And by adding a few natural grains and seeds, you can increase the food value and still keep the calorie level down.

Chapter Six

Delicious Diet Lunches

Your allowable calories for lunch will naturally depend on the total amount you are allocated each day and also on whether you are on three or six meals a day. For most people, however, lunch is generally the smallest meal of the day. Even those who are not trying to lose weight will often have a light lunch; a big meal invariably makes one feel sluggish, something to avoid in the middle of the day; so dieting or not, make lunch an adequate but small meal.

You will not be over or under-extending yourself if you think about lunch in terms of around 300 calories, unless, of course, you are on the 800 a day total! But with 800-1200 calories a day, a lunch of 300 calories is realistic, and with proper planning, you can have a very satisfying and nutritious meal within these limits.

If you are a sandwich-fiend, you can still have your favorite kind, but slightly modified. The typical delicatessen sandwich is *out;* most of these run anywhere from 600 to 1000 calories alone! But watching the type of bread and the thickness of the slice will help keep your sandwich within acceptable limits.

French, Italian or Boston Brown breads run over 100 calories a slice. Cracked wheat, raisin and white run around 60. Whole wheat and rye are your best bets: around 55 calories a regular slice, so slice it thin and cut down even more! Bread made from low-starch flour ("gluten" bread) contains only 35 calories a slice. So vary between low-starch and whole wheat and you'll have variety plus low calories. And rather than have two slices, you can use several of the open-face varieties which need only one slice of bread. We have several recipes for such dishes a little further on.

For those of you who prefer rolls, we advise strictly open-face, as most rolls run around 150 calories. Half is still 75, more than a slice of bread, so this may mean cutting down in other areas.

For filling your sandwich, we advise you to buy your own beef or ham, cook it, and slice it yourself. This will work out much cheaper than buying the packaged cold cuts, and also keeps those extra chemicals out of your body. Pre-packaged cold meats are usually heavily laden with artificial color and preservatives. Also, by cooking your own, you can minimize the fat content by cutting off the excess. Boiled ham works out to only 198 calories for three ounces, with roast ham, turkey or beef, even less: 138 calories! And if you have a meat grinder, you can utilize those small pieces you cut off to make ground cooked filler for shepherd pie and meat loaf, recipes for which are included in a later chapter.

If you prefer a hamburger for lunch, remember the leaner the meat, the fewer the calories. A three ounce hamburger from many restaurants or made from packaged hamburger tips the caloric scale at 245. Having your own pure lean beef ground to order (or grinding it yourself) will give you a three ounce hamburger with only 185 calories. And don't forget: Broil it, don't fry! And broil under a low flame, gently, so as not to scorch the outside.

Cheese is a popular low-calorie luncheon staple, from the now legendary cottage cheese and peaches to many other variations. For those who enjoy this dish, we recommend it highly: 3 ounces of cottage cheese is only 75 calories, and one fresh peach sliced, 35, making a total of only 110 calories. Together with a small fresh green salad, this will give you bulk, nourishment and good balanced food value and still keep you well within a reasonable caloric limit.

For those who enjoy cream cheese but hesitate because of the calories (55 per tablespoon), try a good substitute: Neufchâtel cheese, with only 37 calories a tablespoon, or Farmer cheese, a spreadable creamy cheese with 27 calories a tablespoon.

Cheese can be added in small cubes to a tossed green salad for added food value, and the variety of cheeses makes for a wide selection of possible salads to tempt you for lunch.

Many single items, such as hard-boiled eggs, cold meats (ham, beef, poultry, fish) and chopped up raw vegetables can be made more appealing by the addition of mayonnaise, but remember that regular mayonnaise contains 100 calories a tablespoon. Low-calorie bottled items provide less, but why not make your own? Here is a recipe for mayonnaise, using only natural ingredients, and we guarantee the flavor will never let you suspect its low calories!

Melt two tablespoons of margarine over a low flame, blend in half a cup of whole wheat flour, stirring well. Then add one cup of water, bring to a slow boil and stir continuously until the mixture thickens. Now add: 2 egg yolks; one cup of vegetable oil (preferably safflower or peanut) ; 2 teaspoons fresh lemon juice; 2 teaspoons vinegar; ½ cup honey; 1 teaspoon sea salt; ½ teaspoon dry mustard; ¼ teaspoon cayenne. These ingredients should be blended first, then added to the hot mixture, slowly, a little at a time, using an electric mixer on slow speed. Once all the ingredients are well mixed, turn up the speed and beat for a minute. Cool and refrigerate, and when completely cold, whip the electric mixer at high speed for another minute. Keep the mayonnaise in the refrigerator in a covered bottle or container. This recipe is not only healthful, containing no chemicals or preservatives, but works out to approximately 55-60 calories a tablespoon. Delicious for dieters!

Another taste trick for raw green salads is to mix in one tablespoon of the following mixture: cottage cheese, yogurt, mustard and a few drops of Worcestershire sauce (you can vary the amounts to your own taste preference). This can often remove the psychological aversion that some people have to eating raw salads, giving a creamy richness that tickles the taste buds without adding a great many calories.

For a truly delicious luncheon dish that totals around 250 calories, try the following: Chop two ounces of lean ham (or for smoother consistency, put through a meat grinder) and blend with one hard-boiled egg, chopped, and one tablespoon each of chopped onion and chopped celery and the mayonnaise recipe given above. For tangier flavor, a few drops of Tabasco or Worcestershire sauce may be added. Spread on one thin slice of whole wheat bread.

A variation of this recipe is the following: 1 ounce of chopped (or ground) cooked ham; 1 ounce Swiss cheese; 1 tablespoon shredded lettuce; 1 small chopped beet; 1 tablespoon chopped onion; 1 tablespoon mayonnaise (your own). Combine the ingredients in a small bowl, stirring thoroughly. You may grate the cheese if you wish, or cut into small pieces. Spread over one slice whole wheat bread. Total calories: about 250.

Our home-made health food mayonnaise is great for tunaburgers. These are a summer favorite, served cold, or if you prefer, the tuna may be warmed first or grilled under the broiler. Take one 6½ ounce can of water-packed tuna and combine with ¼ cup of natural mayonnaise and ¼ cup finely chopped celery. Spread on one half a hamburger roll or a slice of whole wheat bread, and sprinkle with a little relish. Real tasty—and each serving gives you only around 145 calories.

Lovers of rye bread will go for this one: Take

one 3½ ounce can of water-packed tuna, drain and mix with 2 tablespoons of yogurt, ½ teaspoon prepared mustard, 2 small mashed beets and ½ teaspoon of chopped fresh parsley. Spread over a slice of rye with one piece of lettuce and sprinkle with paprika. Around 200 calories and really taste-tempting.

Of course there are always those who prefer a hot sandwich or a hot dish for lunch, and in the winter this makes good sense. Warmth as well as nourishment can make a pleasant break in the middle of a chilly day. We've already talked about hamburgers and the variety of this dish is limited only by your imagination. As one example, a tablespoon of finely chopped onion mixed with your three ounces of lean meat, plus a shake of Worcestershire sauce, makes an especially appetizing change, and topping this with natural imitation sour cream only makes the entire dish add up to 220 calories.

You might question "natural imitation" sour cream, which does sound like a contradiction! However, the natural refers to the ingredients, and the imitation to the item, made as follows: ¼ cup of cottage cheese; 1 tablespoon buttermilk, combined by hand-stirring or in a mixer. A teaspoon of this on top of the onion-hamburger or on a salad makes a big taste difference.

California is notorious for its variety of food items, one of which is the famous Pizzaburger, a real zingy luncheon item that contains 280 calories—maybe a little more than your diet calls for, but if you can afford it, this dish makes a welcome change: Broil your hamburger as usual, using two ounces instead of three. Place on a piece of whole wheat or rye bread and top with a mixture of 1 ounce of part skim mozzarella cheese, 1 tablespoon catsup and ¼ teaspoon of oregano. Place under the broiler until it begins to bubble. Remove and serve.

A Bombayburger is another exotic variation: Blend three ounces of lean meat with ¼ teaspoon curry powder and ¼ teaspoon chopped onion. Broil as usual and serve on whole wheat bread topped with a slice of crushed fresh peach and a slice of banana. Scrumptious—and only 220 calories. Go easy with the curry powder, however; too much is liable to blow the top of your head off!

For Western fans, the El Diabloburger will satisfy your craving for barbecue with only 220 calories: Broil three ounces of lean meat as usual, then add the following sauce: 1/3 cup tomato sauce (or fresh tomatoes liquefied in a blender); 1/3 teaspoon fresh lemon juice; 1 teaspoon finely chopped fresh onion; a shake of Worcestershire sauce and a pinch of dry mustard. Bring to a gentle boil and add one teaspoon honey. Stir thoroughly and spoon over the meat, served on whole wheat bread.

Turkey or chicken make excellent bases for a hot luncheon item. Place one slice of chicken or turkey on a piece of whole wheat bread, top with ½ an ounce of grated cheddar cheese and pop under the broiler until the cheese melts. Sprinkle with chopped onion or parsley and a shake of paprika. Around 260 calories per serving.

Of course, your choice of a luncheon dish should begin with the total luncheon calories, and if you desire several items (main dish, salad and fruit, perhaps) start by subtracting the calories from the smaller items from the total to give you the maximum allowable for the main dish. Or merely select whatever appeals to you and add up the calories, which works very well for those who make lunch a combination of small items, such as one hard-boiled egg, one small salad, one apple, and so on. The final decision is naturally up to your own preference, but we feel one main dish, however small or low in calories, offers the psychological satisfaction of having had a meal rather than a snack.

We stress again that psychological attitude is vital. With every meal, in fact with everything you put into your stomach, you must maintain the positive feeling that you are working towards a definite goal of weight loss. Too many people fall into the trap of thinking that just a little extra here and there won't matter; *everything* matters, from that small piece of candy to an extra piece of fruit. The lunch hour is when many dieters add those extra calories.

There is an obvious reason: Dieters who have had a sparse breakfast, and perhaps nothing since, are experiencing pangs of hunger around lunchtime. There is a natural urge to over-extend one's calories, but if you remind yourself that if you do go over (intentionally or not) you'll only defeat your diet. Dieters need strength and courage. Strength of will and courage to stick to your prescribed maximum calories each day are essential if you're going to get rid of those unwanted pounds.

You can also make dieting more interesting and stimulating to your imagination by inventing your

101

own low-calorie dishes. Cottage cheese is a highly recommended staple in most diets, but we won't deny that many people resist the idea because of prior conditioning. However, cottage cheese can be varied in so many ways to make taste-tempting dishes, from the addition of chopped or mashed fruits to blending with many raw vegetables and spices. A perky combination, for example, is to mix one cup of cottage cheese with chopped bell peppers, chopped chives, alfalfa sprouts and onion—very healthful and certainly spicy! So after you've arrived at your caloric limits, put your imagination to work to make reducing *fun!* As any cook knows, half the excitement of cooking is seeing how the end results turn out; the same applies to choosing various items to maintain appetite interest in the many different dishes you can include in your menu.

Many of the recipes in later chapters can be used either for luncheon or dinner dishes, or varied to suit the particular meal. The meat loaf or casserole-type dish forms a good item for dinner, but a slice of meat loaf or shepherd pie can also be good for lunch. Also, the roasts can be used for a multitude of other dishes: sliced cold meats for sandwiches; fried in a whole-wheat batter for another hot dish; the small pieces used for hash; and so on.

From a protein standpoint, as well as calories, roast beef, lamb, pork or veal can work out to be economical both for the budget and the waistline because of the variety of uses to which a cooked roast can be put. Imagination, a little effort and perhaps some spices or a sauce can transform leftovers into sparkling new menu magic.

We mentioned before that liver is one of the most highly recommended sources of natural protein, plus vitamins and minerals. While not every family claps its hands over liver for dinner (there seems to be an undeniable minority of liver fans), the dieter can include liver as a luncheon dish, suitably cooked natural-style to add flavor and taste. Beef liver should be fried fat-free (lecithin or a little vegetable oil may be used on a non-stick skillet) and barely three minutes on each side; just until the meat has turned brown, with the darker patches across the surface. Slice half an onion and half an apple, and chop together finely, then saute in a teaspoon of butter or vegetable oil and serve over the top of the liver. Delicious and only 140 calories, using 3 ounces of liver. Be certain not to overcook liver; this will destroy not only a lot of the natural goodness, but also flavor and tenderness. Also, do not sprinkle salt over liver before or during cooking; this will draw out the juices and minimize its flavor, as well as making it tough. Add salt to your taste at the table.

Chicken livers au naturel are great for lunch. Take half a pound of fresh chicken livers, roll in wheat germ and cook in one tablespoon of vegetable oil over medium heat for about ten minutes, or until nicely brown. Stir in ¼ cup chopped onion, chopped peppers and a dash of sweet basil; cook for two minutes, covered. Making two servings at 160 calories each, this dish is very good with a small green salad and whole wheat bread, all of which will still bring you in under the 300 calorie limit.

The above chicken liver dish can also be put

through a meat grinder after it has been cooled, then stirred or mashed to form a home-made liverwurst that is excellent for sandwiches or snacks. It will keep in the refrigerator in a covered jar. You can also make your own beef liverwurst, which makes a great sandwich on whole wheat bread with a sprinkling of alfalfa sprouts instead of lettuce.

Leftover pieces of chicken or ham can also be put through a meat grinder to make a *pate;* a few drops of Worcestershire sauce or Tabasco (depending on your preference) and you have a tasty sandwich spread, low in calories and a lot cheaper than the canned variety.

Many people complain that a dieter's sandwich is often dry, unless laced with mayonnaise. If you can't afford the calories in mayonnaise, try having a cup of bouillon with your sandwich. This will provide liquid, warmth and minimal calories. Home-made bouillon or the dehydrated type in granulated form gives only 5-10 calories per cupful, either beef, chicken, onion or vegetable. Bouillon also makes a great mid-morning or afternoon snack, filling and fortifying without upsetting the caloric apple-cart!

Soups are also excellent for lunch, especially home-made natural soups, and we go into these in a later chapter with recipes that give you a complete meal in a soupbowl for less than 300 calories. These hearty soups are very good psychologically, because, for whatever reason, they seem to be more filling than many other dishes, giving you the feeling of having had a hearty meal and leaving you with a truly satisfied stomach.

Lunch can often be a problem for working people. Plan ahead: Just as there is no sense starving yourself at breakfast, lunch should be a break that provides you with sufficient nourishment to continue through the day. Skipping lunch only means you're going to automatically want to eat more at dinner and perhaps over-extend yourself on your caloric limit. So plan your schedule and stick to it.

Chapter Seven

Dinner Main Courses

Traditionally, dinner is the largest meal of the day and also one many of us look forward to most of all. Pre-conditioning plays such a role in our eating habits; instinctively we anticipate a major meat dish with several vegetables, plus perhaps a soup to start with and a goopy dessert to finish off the meal. For a dieter, dinner can be murder! But—it doesn't have to be. By careful choice of ingredients, closer attention to cooking and keeping calories in mind, you can have a mouthwatering spread that every member of the family will enjoy without even being aware that it is low-calorie.

It is often psychologically devastating when only one member of a family is on a diet, because of the separation of food items. The dieter sits down, surrounded by temptation, with only some raw carrots, celery and a few crackers on his own plate.

By cooking naturally and low-calorically, not only will a person with a restricted diet benefit, but every member of the family will as well; for it is generally known that we eat too much, especially at dinner. So cutting down on the calories for everyone will improve the entire family's health. The recipes that follow include just as much flavor and taste-appeal as ordinary cooking, plus the added nutrition that natural ingredients contribute. This is of particular significance in families with teenagers. Establishing a well-balanced menu for growing youngsters can help them avoid weight problems in their mature years and give them a healthy start in life, not only physically but mentally as well. If kids are taught good eating habits during the growing years, these will remain and form a foundation for their attitude towards diet as adults. Far too many children grow up with the "coke-and-hamburger" syndrome or the "malt-and-hot-dog" routine after school, which plays havoc with their regular mealtime appetites as well as their general metabolism.

A main meat or fish dish for dinner will provide the basic protein that is essential in everyone's daily diet. Whatever form the meat or fish takes, take care in the preparation not to waste the natural ingredients or destroy the food value through improper cooking.

As a general rule, meat benefits from undercooking rather than over-cooking. Even pork, which has to be thoroughly cooked as a precaution against possible disease in hogs, need not be burned to a crisp as so often happens. There is a difference between *cooked* and *over-cooked*. A meat thermometer is useful for determining when the inside of a roast is done to the desired degree, although many experienced cooks can tell from appearance and cooking time.

We recommend roasts because of their versatility and fringe benefits. And in spite of the rising cost, meat is still a bargain, considering the food value; and if you plan ahead, you can make one large roast come out more economically than ground meat! This is a fact: A large rolled roast, for example, serves as one meal in its original state. Slices provide luncheon meats for sandwiches. The small pieces lost in carving can be saved and added to the final pieces to make a shepherd pie, which in turn can be sliced for sandwiches as well as hot luncheon dishes. Imagination plus planning will enable you to cook better and more economically.

If you are a country cousin rather than a city dweller, you may well benefit by buying your meat in bulk from a farmer, which gives you naturally raised beef over the usual mass-produced products that can sometimes have unacceptable additives in the cattle feed. We are not saying that supermarket beef is to be avoided. Far from it; but if you can get your meat from a farmer, you will get a cheaper and more nutritious selection for your freezer. You would also be well advised to seek out a butcher where you can be sure of top quality meat, cut to your specification, rather than take the cellophane-wrapped variety in most supermarkets. Smaller butchers invariably will give you better value as they are eager to keep their customers, who will only come back if they are satisfied, both in the cut and the way it is trimmed. By trimming, we naturally mean cutting off the fat, which doesn't do any good except add calories.

We refer you back to the description of the various grades of beef, too: Remember that all grades of meat are equally nutritious, but the cheaper ones require a different approach in cooking to insure tenderness. Top quality may be good for oven roasts, but the lower grades are quite acceptable for dishes where cooking time and method brings out flavor and tenderness. Many restaurants boast of "ground sirloin"—which is admittedly good; but ground beef is ground beef, and once it goes through the grinder, the cut makes little difference. A chat to your butcher will prove beneficial in selecting the cuts that give you the best value for your money. Remember, he may well try to disparage your taking a lower grade because naturally he wants to sell the higher priced item, which is only good business. But don't be put off; if you plan meat loaf or a casserole, get the cheapest grade you can, have it trimmed properly, then cut into very small pieces, marinate in your favorite sauce and simmer gently, then proceed with your recipe as usual. You'll save in money and calories. For example one pound of rib steak (meat only) is 45 percent fat and more than 2,000 calories. Fat-trimmed, lean, round pot roast is less than 700 calories per pound.

Using natural food items in your dinners can result in very adequate meals for the entire family; the dieter merely has to restrict his amount in proportion to the amount of calories allocated for the meal. A dieter may have, for example, only one slice of meat, two vegetables and a piece of fruit; but the rest of the family can have three or four slices and as many vegetables as they desire. Everyone is happy and the dieter still feels his diet has not become a burden for the cook!

Pot Roasts

Again: Steak is *not* the most advisable dish for a dieter, both from a caloric standpoint as well as cost. A slow-simmered pot roast can be less than half the calories. Chuck and flank steaks are also ideal for dieting menus. Don't forget that the more fat you eliminate by trimming meat, the less saturated fats you will have in the final dish. Here is a list of some common cuts of boneless uncooked beef with their fat content and calories listed for comparison:

	Fat Content	Calories Per Pound
Flank Steak	0%	650
Round Steak	11%	890
Chuck Arm	14%	1000
Rump, Roundbone Sirloin, Doublebone Sirloin, Blade Steak, Chuck Rib	25-30%	1300-1500
Club Steak	36%	1700
Porterhouse, T-Bone, Hipbone Sirloin	37-39%	1700-1800
Short Plate	41%	1800
Rib (11th and 12th)	45%	2000

Chuck and flank steaks can give you low calories and low cost, and with care, can provide all the flavor and tenderness you are accustomed to from higher priced (and higher caloried!) cuts.

Of the six grades listed earlier, the top three are usually available at most butchers; the lowest three are held for commercial use, but this doesn't mean you can't get them if you talk to your butcher. Remember that grade and cut affect the fat content of beef. Cuts from the hind quarter of the animal are less fatty than cuts from the front part of the carcass.

As pot roast is a recommended method of cooking meat to minimize fat and conserve flavor, we suggest you plan ahead for this dish. After trimming and marinating (if desired), brown and simmer the meat by itself, then refrigerate overnight in the same pot. Next day, skim off the hardened fat from the top and continue cooking, adding the vegetables and, before serving, making your sauce or gravy (using arrowroot, not flour) and you'll have a low-calorie, delicious roast that will rate raves at the dinner table.

In browning the meat, as with *any* dish included in a low-calorie menu, use only one tablespoon of vegetable oil, and after browning, drain off any fat in the pot before continuing. No matter how carefully you trim off every bit of fat, there will naturally always be some that accumulates during the browning stage.

Alternatively, you can brown the meat under the broiler, which is even better, allowing any fat to drain off into the drip pan. If you usually use these scrapings for gravy, instead use soy sauce, Worcestershire sauce or a dash of a commercial gravy powder (such as Bisto) for the final savory touch.

Many people cannot resist cooking vegetables in the fatty drippings from a pot roast. Forget this idea; vegetables soak up fat quicker than paper towels! Steam your vegetables or use a double boiler and let them cook in their own juices—far healthier and better tasting!

Lean meats naturally take longer to cook than a usual fatty cut, anywhere from 25 to 50 percent longer in the pot. Don't try to hurry a pot roast; high heat will only make the meat tough, and you wind up with wasted effort and wasted food. Slow, steady simmering brings out the best in any meat, particularly the cheaper cuts. Turn your flame down to the lowest possible level and use a good pot, preferably stainless steel waterless cookware which requires minimum heat and helps keep the vapors from escaping.

Another point to remember: The leaner the beef, the less the loss through shrinkage. A lean boneless pot roast, properly simmered very slowly, can give you three to four three-ounce servings per pound, making it truly economical.

Here is a good basic recipe for pot roast, using round steak, which is only 11 percent fat and 890 calories per pound. The amount is for 12 three-ounce servings, giving you plenty for a family meal, plus enough left over for slices for sandwiches and another meal off the same roast. Start with 3½ pounds of round steak, well-trimmed and lean. Season with garlic salt, pepper and rub all over with Worcestershire sauce and prepared mustard. Place a tablespoon of vegetable oil in a large Dutch oven, preferably stainless steel or non-stick coated, and heat until very hot. Lower the meat in, turning quickly to cover all sides with the hot oil. Continue cooking until all sides are browned. Drain off the oil, lower the heat and add the following: one bay leaf; one teaspoon crumbled leaf thyme; one teaspoon brown sugar; two cups of beef bouillon. Cover and simmer over very low heat for three hours. The liquid should not bubble rapidly, but barely boil, allowing the meat to cook gently. You can check it every hour to make sure the liquid is not boiling away; you can add another cup of bouillon if necessary after an hour or two.

Remove from the stove, take out the bay leaf, and refrigerate overnight. An hour before your dinner time, take out the pot and scrape off any solidified fat from the top of the liquid. Add two chopped onions and two tablespoons of chopped parsley. Place on low flame and simmer for about forty-five minutes.

Take out the meat and if you prefer a thick gravy, add arrowroot to the liquid and allow to boil briefly; or serve the gravy as is: thin, but tasty and nutritious. Each three-ounce serving contains 205 calories.

For those who like a gourmet touch without the gourmet calories, here is a variation on pot roast that has its roots in an old French country dish, complete with wine for flavor. (Wine loses its calories in cooking but not its taste.)

This recipe also uses round steak, starting with 3 pounds, seasoned with garlic salt, pepper, Worcestershire sauce and prepared mustard as in the preceding instructions. Again use only a tablespoon of vegetable oil, heated in a large Dutch oven until very hot. Brown the meat, pour off the oil, then add the following ingredients: ½ cup dry red wine; ½ cup beef bouillon; 16 ounces of tomato sauce or fresh tomatoes that you have liquefied in a blender; 1 bay leaf. Simmer for three hours, over a very low flame. Check every hour to make sure there is plenty of liquid, and add another cup of bouillon if necessary. Remove from the stove and refrigerate overnight. An hour before serving, skim the hardened fat from the top, and add half a cup of chopped onion and one cup of shredded carrots (or small whole ones). Simmer for half an hour over a low flame, with the pot covered, as it should be in the initial cooking.

Before serving, remove the meat and, if desired, thicken the gravy, though this particular gravy is fairly thick by itself and very delicious, especially when served over rice.

Another French dish, slightly modified by the Dutch and presently popular in the Cape section of South Africa, also calls for wine in the cooking and contains only about 240 calories for a three ounce serving.

Prepare 3½ pounds of lean, well-trimmed round steak as in the two preceding recipes. After browning and pouring off the oil, add the following ingredients: 1 teaspoon poultry seasoning; 1 teaspoon pumpkin-pie spice; ½ teaspoon grated orange rind; ½ teaspoon grated lemon rind; 2 teaspoons parsley flakes (or chopped fresh parsley); 1 cup sliced onion; 1 cup sliced carrots; 1 cup sliced mushrooms (fresh); ½ cup Burgundy wine; 2½ cups beef bouillon. Simmer very gently for three hours. Remove and refrigerate overnight. An hour before serving, skim off the fat from the top, place back on the stove over a low flame and simmer for a half hour. Remove the meat, and thicken the gravy with 2 tablespoons of arrowroot or cornstarch, bringing to a quick boil and then taking it off the stove.

There are many variations of pot roast, but the eternal favorite seems to be the traditional New England recipe. However, again we stress the usual method of cooking means calorie-laden meat *and* vegetables, so follow the following directions and you'll be serving the traditional dish in a modern way, meaning fewer calories. Although we use chuck, which is richer than round steak, removing the fat after initial cooking brings it down to a dieter's level: only 240 calories per three ounce serving.

Start off with 3½ pounds of chuck arm roast, boneless and trimmed of all fat. The leaner the better! Season only with salt and pepper, and brown in a tablespoon of vegetable oil, pouring off the oil after all sides are brown. Add three cups of beef bouillon; 2 bay leaves; 1 teaspoon poultry seasoning; simmer gently for three hours. Refrigerate overnight.

Half an hour before dinner time, remove the hardened fat from the top, and place on the stove over a low flame. Add three large stalks of celery, scraped and cut into six inch lengths; four large carrots, scraped and sliced lengthwise, eight small onions, peeled; two turnips, peeled and cut in slices. Simmer until the vegetables are done, usually about 20 minutes. Remove the meat and thicken the gravy with 2 tablespoons of cornstarch or arrowroot, allowing to boil briefly, then serve. If you find the flavor too bland, you can always perk it up by adding two teaspoons of Worcestershire sauce, though New England pot roast is traditionally bland.

Half the fun of cooking naturally is experimenting with dishes that are new to your menu: And even pot roast takes on a fresh twist when you change it from New England to France—or China or Italy! Try the following two recipes for something deliciously different—*and* low caloried, too!

Those of you who have already started growing your own sprouts will welcome this version of pot roast, sometimes called Shanghai Pot Roast. Again we start out with boneless, well-trimmed chuck arm roast, 3½ pounds, seasoned with salt and pepper, then rubbed well all over with soy sauce and allowed to stand for a half hour. Then brown in a tablespoon of vegetable oil, drain, and then add the following: one cup dry sherry; one cup beef bouillon; 5 tablespoons soy sauce; 1 teaspoon ground ginger; ¼ teaspoon pepper; 1 teaspoon dry mustard; ½ teaspoon sweet basil. Simmer gently for 3 hours, then refrigerate overnight.

An hour before serving, skim the solidified fat from the top and place back on a low flame. Take one large onion and, together with a tablespoon of water, liquefy in a blender (or you can chop it yourself, very fine). When the liquid is simmering, add the onions, plus two cups of sprouts, whichever variety you prefer. Bean sprouts are usually best or you may use a complete mixture of Chinese vegetables instead, which include bean sprouts, as well as water chestnuts and peapods. Allow to cook gently for 20 minutes, then serve. The gravy and vegetable mixture is especially good over rice, or if you prefer (and your diet can stand it!), noodles. You can also use the second half of this recipe (the vegetable portion) for perking up a left-over New England style pot roast. Whatever meat is left from a previous meal is merely warmed in its own gravy, then the vegetable mixture is added. Simmer 20 minutes before serving.

From China to Italy—in only 210 calories per three ounce serving. This dish is tasty, spicy and, since flank steak is used, economical.

You will need 1½ pounds of flank steak, sliced on the thin side, not more than ½ inch thick. Make several crosscuts about halfway through the meat, turn over and spread with the following: 2 tablespoons grated Romano cheese; 1 teaspoon oregano; 1 teaspoon garlic salt; ¼ teaspoon pepper. Now roll into a long sausage shape and tie firmly every couple of inches with fine string or white twine. Nylon thread is also good, wrapped around and around to enclose the meat in its sausage-shape.

Place 1 tablespoon olive oil in a deep pan or Dutch oven and heat fairly hot. Drop the meat in, and roll around until it is well browned on all sides. Drain off the oil. Now add the following ingredients: 1 pound of fresh tomatoes that have been liquefied in a blender after removing the skins; 1 cup of water; ¼ teaspoon oregano; ¼ teaspoon pepper; 1 onion that has been liquefied in the blender (at the same time as the tomatoes). Cover and simmer gently for 2 hours. Remove the meat and place on a serving platter. Cook the sauce a while longer until thick; or you may add a little arrowroot to thicken it, but be careful with your heat, so that the sauce does not stick to the bottom of the pan and burn. Pour the sauce over the meat after removing the string. Slice cross-wise for individual servings. This amount should serve 6 persons, each with a three-ounce portion.

Shepherd Pie

This recipe requires that you have your own meat grinder, as the main constituent consists of ground-up leftover pieces of meat from roasts. Trim off any pieces of fatty tissue that may remain; the meat going into the grinder must be all lean.

Once you have all your leftover, cooked meat ground up, place in a bowl and add one egg, salt and pepper and a dash of Worcestershire sauce. Stir until thoroughly mixed; then spread over the bottom of a conveniently-sized casserole. You should have enough meat to cover the bottom at least by about two inches; if you don't have enough meat, use a small casserole.

Take one large onion and chop finely; spread over the top of the meat. Now cover the top with firmly mashed potatoes. If you wish, you can make an interesting design on the mashed potatoes with a fork.

Pop in a hot oven (350-375 degrees) for 30 minutes, or until the potatoes are crisply browned. Before serving, add a sprinkle of chopped parsley mixed with bean sprouts. Delicious! We might add that if you are using a glass casserole, rather than the Corningware type, it is advisable to stand it in a pan of water to prevent cracking and also to keep the meat moist. Shepherd pie can be served hot as a main dish, or sliced the next day for sandwiches, open-faced and warmed. Depending upon the thickness of the meat and the mashed potato topping, one serving contains approximately 150 calories.

Stew and Curry

Many dieters automatically look on stews as

fattening, which they need not be: Take the following recipe, which contains only 220 calories per serving: Start with 2 pounds of trimmed, boneless round steak, as lean as you can get it, and cut into small cubes—the smaller the better. Place a cup of wheat germ in a paper bag, put in your pieces of meat and shake well, holding your hand underneath to give some support.

Have a large Dutch oven ready with a tablespoon of vegetable oil, heated fairly hot. Take your pieces of beef, now nicely coated with the wheat germ, and put in the pot, stirring rapidly with a spoon. By the time each piece has browned, the oil should have all been absorbed in the wheat germ coating, giving you a dry pot with the meat seared nicely.

Add: 1 cup of sherry; 2 cups of beef bouillon; 1 cup of diced carrots; 2 large sliced onions; 1 cup sliced mushrooms; ½ cup chopped celery; ½ cup green peas; ½ teaspoon sea salt; ¼ teaspoon pepper; 1 teaspoon Worcestershire sauce; ½ teaspoon garlic salt. Bring to a boil, then turn the heat down and simmer very gently for 2 hours. Allow to cool, and refrigerate overnight. Next day, simmer for another hour before serving, by which time your stew should be rich and fairly thick. If you prefer a thicker consistency, add a teaspoon or two of cornstarch or arrowroot.

For a spicy difference, you may turn the above stew into a beef curry by merely adding two teaspoons of curry powder 30 minutes before serving. For those who like it really hot, more curry powder may be added, but be sure and test it by taste first. That curry powder can be dynamite to your digestion!

Both the stew or the curry may be served over

white or brown rice, together with a quick-n-easy chutney made from half a cup of apricot jam and a tablespoon of Worcestershire sauce.

Enriching Ground Beef

Many meat dishes can be upped in protein value by adding items like wheat germ to the original recipe. One in particular that is easy to make and very good for perking up jaded appetites is low-calorie beef balls stroganoff.

Take two pounds of the leanest ground beef you can get (or, as recommended, grind your own) and combine this in a bowl with the whites of two eggs. (We would like to stress that in binding meat, use only the whites. Yolks only add unnecessary calories and are not needed for binding.) Add the following: ½ cup finely chopped fresh onion; ½ cup wheat germ; 1 teaspoon prepared mustard. Mix together thoroughly.

Take about a dessert spoon of the meat mixture and roll into a ball, then roll in wheat germ. Continue until all the meat is rolled in balls, then place in a wide skillet that has been sprayed with lecithin. Cook over a low flame until the meat balls are browned on all sides (usually around five minutes). Place on one side.

Combine the following ingredients in a bowl: 2 cups of beef bouillon; ½ teaspoon sea salt; ¼ teaspoon pepper; 1 teaspoon Worcestershire sauce; 1 teaspoon mustard; 1 teaspoon chopped parsley (or parsley flakes); 1 cup finely chopped mushrooms (fresh or canned); ¼ teaspoon sweet basil. Blend and pour over the browned meat balls, replace over heat and simmer gently for 30 minutes. Take out the meat balls and place in a serving dish. Now add to the pot: ¼ cup sherry; 1 cup yogurt (or buttermilk); 1 tablespoon kelp. Allow to simmer for one minute only. Remove and pour over the meat balls, and serve. This recipe makes 8-10 servings of around 170 calories each.

Ordinary meat patties (we call them that because they're thicker than hamburgers) can be enriched with protein by adding the following mixture to a pound of lean ground round: 1 cup high-protein cereal or grains; ½ cup skim milk; ¼ teaspoon powdered sage; 4 tablespoons minced onion; 1 egg white; 3 teaspoons granulated beef bouillon. Mix together well, shape into four patties and broil gently until cooked to the desired degree. One pound gives you 4 patties of 230 calories each. An enriched patty makes a tasty and nourishing main dish for lunch, as well as being a good main dinner course. These patties can also be used to prepare a traditional beef-and-eggplant Greek dish that adds only 50 calories per serving.

Cook your four patties as above, then cut them into bite-sized chunks. Place in a deep baking dish, together with 1 eggplant, pared and sliced into cubes. Cover with 16 ounces of liquefied fresh tomatoes (or tomato sauce) into which you have stirred 2 tablespoons of minced fresh onion, 2 teaspoons garlic salt, ¼ teaspoon nutmeg and a pinch of sea salt. Sprinkle with 2 tablespoons of grated cheese. Cover with foil and bake in a moderate oven (350 degrees) for 30 minutes. Remove the foil and bake another 30 minutes, or until the eggplant is tender. Serve with a little extra fresh grated cheese on top.

Meat loaf is an old stand-by for most cooks, but this recipe is quite unusual and flavorful—and a favorite for those who cook with natural foods.

You need 1 pound of lean ground beef. Place in a mixing bowl and combine with one egg, stirring thoroughly. Now add the following: 2 fresh tomatoes, liquefied in a blender, after removing the skins; 2 teaspoons fresh chopped parsley; ½ cup wheat germ; ¼ cup soy grits that have been soaked in ½ cup of water; 1 finely chopped onion; 1 teaspoon corn oil; 1 teaspoon fresh lemon juice; 1 teaspoon sweet basil; 1 teaspoon tarragon. Mix thoroughly and place in a small loaf pan or casserole that has been sprayed with lecithin to prevent the meat from sticking. Bake in a moderate oven (350 degrees) for one hour. May be served hot with a salad or fresh green vegetables, or sliced cold the next day for sandwiches. One fairly thin slice totals out to a little under 100 calories.

A great low-calorie beef and green vegetable loaf will give you six servings at only 170 calories each. Use one pound of very lean ground round and mix together with the following items: 1 cup of creamed style cottage cheese; 4 tablespoons wheat germ; 1 cup of shredded fresh carrots; ¼ cup chopped fresh onion; 1 egg white; 1 teaspoon sea salt; ½ teaspoon sweet basil; ¼ teaspoon pepper. Place in a 9 inch round cake pan and shape into a circular loaf. Bake in a moderate oven (350 degrees) for about 45 minutes, or until the loaf is firm and browned on top. Allow to cool for about ten minutes before cutting it with a very sharp knife.

Most vegetables can be utilized to expand a meat loaf-type recipe, and the more natural vegetables you use, the greater will be the nutritional value of the dish. Although the usual spices and herbs used to enhance flavor contribute little in calories, the taste of good fresh vegetables can often be a welcome change. Sprouts, chopped string beans, peas, diced eggplant, are all excellent additions to meat loaf. Experiment yourself to determine which appeals most to your family's tastebuds, and whenever you can, add some wheat germ to the recipe for extra protein and a rich, nutty flavor.

A rich natural topping for ground round patties can be made as follows: Combine 2 tablespoons margarine with two teaspoons of wheat germ; 1/4 teaspoon garlic salt; 4 tablespoons chopped parsley; 1/4 teaspoon grated lemon rind; 1 teaspoon lemon juice. Broil your ground round patties until almost done, then top each one with the mixture and replace under the broiler for about 2-3 minutes, or until bubbly and browning. Remove and serve. For each 1/4 pound of ground round cooked like this, you chalk up only 160 calories!

Beef Kidney

The English have a traditional dish, steak and kidney pie, in which the amount of kidney used is just enough to enhance the overall flavor. The same principle can be applied to meat loaf: adding about 1/4 cup of chopped, cooked kidneys to a meat loaf recipe calling for one pound of ground beef. The addition results in a different zesty flavor, plus added nutrition. Kidneys are also excellent cooked with liver and bacon as a main dinner dish.

Veal

Veal is one of the lowest calorie meats you can buy and, as such, is a good addition to a dieter's menu. Although some people object to the blandness of veal compared with beef, this meat can form the basis for many taste-tempting dishes, especially when perked up with fruit and spices, like this easy recipe for a sweet and sour Chinese-style dinner which makes about 6 servings at around 275 calories each: Take 1½ pounds of veal shoulder and cut into small cubes; brown in a skillet, using 1 tablespoon vegetable oil. Add: one cup beef bouillon; ½ cup finely chopped onion; 1 medium-sized can of pineapple chunks, including the juice; simmer for 45 minutes.

Now add: 1 cup chopped celery; ½ cup bean sprouts; 1 tablespoon wine vinegar; 3 tablespoons soy sauce; 2 teaspoons arrowroot or cornstarch; ½ teaspoon sea salt; a dash of pepper. Simmer gently for ten minutes and serve.

Wine lends itself well to veal dishes; try the following recipe for an impressively rich tasting dish, but with only 260 calories per serving: Cut two pounds of veal shoulder into cubes and brown in 1 tablespoon of vegetable oil. Add: ½ cup chopped onion; 1 minced garlic clove; 1 pound fresh, sliced mushrooms; ½ cup sprouts. Stir gently while cooking until the onion is partly cooked, about three minutes. Add: ¾ cup sherry; 1½ teaspoons sea salt; ½ teaspoon lemon juice; ¼ teaspoon pepper; 1 bay leaf. Simmer gently for 1 hour. Remove bay leaf and serve with a sprinkling of chopped parsley.

Another 260-calorie-per-serving dish: veal rolls Milanese, which look as good as they taste. Use 1½ pounds of veal, sliced thin into 6 or 8 pieces. Cover with the following mixture: 4 ounces chopped ham; 2 hard-boiled eggs, mashed; ½ cup minced onion; 4 tablespoons chopped parsley; 4

tablespoons wheat germ; ½ teaspoon poultry seasoning; 3 tablespoons liquefied fresh tomatoes (without the skins). Spread evenly over the strips of veal and roll up. Tie with twine or nylon thread. Place seam-side-down in a shallow baking dish and brush the tops with a mixture of half olive oil, half fresh lemon juice. Cover and bake in a moderate oven (350 degrees) for 1 hour.

Veal parmigiana is a perennial favorite, but usually tips the calorie scale at 600 per serving! Try this recipe, which cuts the calories in half but does not sacrifice that sought-after flavor: Use 1½ pounds of thinly sliced veal. Dip the pieces in wheat germ and brown briefly in 1 tablespoon olive oil. Place in a shallow baking dish and cover with the following mixture: 16 ounces liquefied fresh tomatoes, skinned; 2 teaspoons oregano; 1 teaspoon garlic salt; ½ teaspoon sea salt; ¼ teaspoon pepper. (Place these in the blender at the same time as you liquefy the tomatoes). Cover with 3 ounces mozzarella cheese, thinly sliced. Bake in a moderate oven (350 degrees) for about 20 minutes, until the cheese topping is bubbling.

Don't overlook veal as a replacement for beef in meat loaf. And leftovers from a veal roast also make a good low-calorie shepherd pie that is particularly good sliced cold for sandwiches.

Lamb

Many people reject lamb because, they claim, it is too fatty. While it is true that lamb chops, no matter which way you cook them, *are* high in calories, lamb has one major advantage over other meats: Unlike beef, where fat is distributed throughout the tissue, lamb fat is mainly on the *outside,* enabling any cook or butcher to trim away the fat, leaving only the lean meat. A leg of lamb, properly trimmed, is the leanest meat, and in our opinion an appealing change from the taste of beef or pork. A leg of lamb is a good low-calorie dish for any dieter, and slices from a raw leg roast make chops that can be broiled or stewed with less calories than the usual type of chop.

So don't sell lamb short. Include it in your menu every week or two. You'll find it acceptable in your diet and an interesting change, like the following shish kebab, which is great for summer barbecues and only 200 calories a serving: Use 1 pound of lean lamb leg, cut into 1 inch squares. Place in a deep bowl and marinate for 2-4 hours in the following mixture: ½ cup water; 1 teaspoon sea salt; 2 teaspoons Worcestershire sauce; ¼ teaspoon thyme; ¼ teaspoon pepper; ½ teaspoon grated lemon rind; 3 tablespoons fresh lemon juice; ¼ teaspoon crushed rosemary; a clove of garlic, pressed.

Spear onto a skewer alternate pieces of meat, tomato wedges, small onions, quartered, and slices of green pepper. Broil, either over charcoal or under the broiler in the oven, for 20 minutes, turning every five minutes and brushing the meat with a little vegetable oil. The meat and vegetables should be nicely browned when ready. Slide off the skewer onto a plate and serve with a tossed salad.

Because of its flavor, lamb is particularly suitable for curry dishes. Try the following recipe for Lamb New Delhi, which gives about 4 servings at 280 calories each. Place in a large saucepan: 1 pound of roast lamb leg, cut into cubes; 3 tablespoons chopped onion; 1 teaspoon garlic salt; 1 teaspoon curry powder; ½ teaspoon ground ginger; 1 teaspoon Worcestershire sauce; 2 cups liquefied fresh tomatoes (beef bouillon can be used instead if you prefer a meatier taste). Simmer for twenty minutes gently. Add arrowroot or cornstarch to thicken slightly. Serve over rice with some crispy broccoli or a vegetable of your choice. To gain a deeper curry flavor for the lamb, you can prepare this dish by browning raw lamb slightly before adding the other ingredients and cooking for two hours. Like all stew-type dishes, this improves with overnight refrigeration and warming up the next day.

Lamb is a legendary favorite in the Middle East, which is where this recipe comes from: possibly the Turkish version of health food meat balls!

Combine in a mixing bowl: 2 pounds of trimmed, raw lamb, freshly ground; 2 eggs; 2 fresh tomatoes, skinned and liquefied; 1 cup chopped parsley; 1½ teaspoons garlic salt; 2 teaspoons brewer's yeast; ½ cup wheat germ; 1 teaspoon cinnamon. Blend together thoroughly and shape into small meatballs about 1-2 inches in diameter. Brown under the broiler or in a non-stick skillet. Place in a deep serving dish and cover with 3 cups of yogurt that has been heated in a double boiler or warmed gently over very low heat; do not allow to boil! Sprinkle with chopped parsley and shower with paprika. Again, beef bouillon can be substituted for the tomato if you prefer a meatier flavor.

For buying lamb, follow these hints: A leg of lamb is highly recommended, provided you get the butcher to trim off *all* fat or, alternatively, have him remove the bone and make up a rolled roast. For barbecue or pan frying, use the lean lamb

127

chops cut from the leg. For stews use the lean portion from the leg, although a shoulder roast, well-trimmed, is a little cheaper and works just as well. For ground lamb, it makes no difference which cut you use, provided the butcher trims off all fat before grinding.

A final taste tip: Lamb in any form goes very well with sliced fried apples, apple sauce, cranberry sauce and, of course, mint sauce or jelly.

Pork

While pork is not the meat known for low calories, many cuts of pork are more than passably suitable for dieters who yearn for this particular dish. Like lamb, pork must be carefully trimmed of all fat to end up with a lean cut that can be temptingly prepared to fit into a low-calorie diet.

Look for the leanest pork you can get from your butcher, forgetting about the marbling so desired in beef; pork has a natural tenderness that does not rely on fatty streaks. Canned hams make a good buy, both for value and low calories, as there is no waste or very little. Forget the traditional glazing and use natural fresh fruit instead; you'll get the same taste tingle without all that sugar! For slow-cooking pork dishes, use boned, trimmed pork shoulder and cook a day ahead, allowing an overnight stay in the refrigerator to bring the fat to the top where it can be skimmed off before reheating, eliminating fats and calories.

A final note: All pork must be thoroughly cooked prior to eating. Using a meat thermometer assures the inside temperature of a roast reaches 170 degrees, the minimum safe level to destroy harmful organisms that may be present.

Here is a tasty recipe for a healthful natural way to prepare pork chops: Place 8 center cut pork chops, ½ inch thick, with all fat trimmed away, in a cold skillet and cook over low heat until browned. (Use a non-stick skillet or spray with lecithin to prevent sticking.) Cover with the following mixture: 2 tablespoons honey; 3 tablespoons orange juice; ½ teaspoon grated orange peel; 1 teaspoon lemon juice; simmer over low heat for 45 minutes. If the liquid becomes too thick, add a *little* water. Remove chops and allow the liquid to simmer until syrupy. Place one slice of orange on top of each chop and cover with syrup. Delicious and only 250 calories.

Pork always seems a stand-by for Chinese cooking. Here's a mock-Chinese recipe that gives six servings at only 190 calories each. Take 1½ pounds of pork steaks, sprinkle with garlic powder and place in a skillet with ½ cup dry sherry and 6 tablespoons of soy sauce. Cover and marinate in the refrigerator for 4 hours, or overnight. Remove the steaks and broil gently, about 12 minutes per side. While the meat is cooking, place the skillet (with the marinade) over a low flame and add the following: 2 skinned fresh tomatoes, liquefied (or ½ cup tomato juice); 1 teaspoon honey; 2 teaspoons cornstarch or arrowroot. Stir until the mixture thickens. Pour over the meat before serving or on the individual portions after slicing.

Most meats get a boost from fruit or vegetables cooked at the same time and pork is no exception. Try this one for a sweet-sour dish that provides 6 servings at around 210 calories each: Place 1½ pounds trimmed pork steak in a skillet with enough water to cover the bottom of the pan.

Cook gently until the water evaporates and the steak browns; turn until the other side is brown as well. Remove the meat and place in the warming oven. Add to the skillet the following items: 1 large can rinsed, drained sauerkraut; 1 cup of chopped onions; 1 cup of apple sauce; ½ teaspoon sea salt; ¼ teaspoon pepper; ½ teaspoon sweet basil. Stir over medium heat, then replace the meat and cook, covered, for about an hour. You may add a little water if the liquid looks like it is evaporating; for a gourmet touch, you may add ¼ cup white wine. Cut into six servings and serve topped with the cooked mixture. This dish is especially good with brown rice and French-style green beans.

Many people have commented that pork, like veal, is too bland a taste compared with beef; however, marinating in various liquids, sauces and herbs can give pork a very interesting flavor, so don't be afraid to experiment with various marinades of your favorite sauces. All you add is flavor, not calories, which makes spiced-up dishes acceptable for dieters as well as the rest of the family. Restricting your calories does not mean losing out on mouth-watering favorites; just let your imagination work overtime!

Chicken

Even with today's higher prices, chicken still constitutes a budget-stretching bargain, both in food value and low calories. A tip for dieters: For chicken dishes that involve cooking in a pot on the stove, rather than baking in the oven, strip off the skin, which is where much of the fat is found. A tablespoon of chicken fat adds around 125 calories—unnecessary in *any* diet! This inherent fat content is what enables you to bake a chicken without adding any oil or butter, which makes chicken with its skin great for roasting. So do not attempt to roast a chicken with the skin removed; you're liable to end up with an unpleasant hard crust.

However, in stews and casseroles, skinned chicken works very well. Skinned chicken can also be used for mock-fried chicken, which means rolling pieces of chicken in bread crumbs or preferably wheat germ and cooking in the oven instead of in fat in a skillet. Whether skinned or not, chicken cooked in the oven (except for casseroles) benefits by covering with aluminum foil to prevent drying out and burning on top.

Although chicken has its own distinctive flavor, the meat is usually helped along by the addition of spices and herbs. In particular, chicken benefits from fruit, as in the following recipe which makes 6 servings at 220 calories each: Use two fryers (about 1½ pounds each), cut up and skinned. Place in a shallow baking dish. Cover with one cup of sliced fresh mushrooms and a sauce made from the following items, simmered over low heat until thick: 1 onion, finely chopped; 1 cup orange juice; 1 teaspoon grated orange peel; 4 tablespoons finely chopped green peppers; 3 tablespoons dry sherry; ½ cup water; 1½ teaspoons sea salt; ½ teaspoon pepper; 2 teaspoons chopped parsley; 1 tablespoon cornstarch, arrowroot or whole wheat flour for thickening.

Bake in moderate oven (350 degrees) for 1-1½ hours, basting frequently. Instead of basting, you may cover the dish with aluminum foil, sealing the edges, for the first 45 minutes of cooking. While the basting method results in improved flavor and better taste throughout the meat, using the foil does free you for other chores.

Baked chicken Hawaiian is an easy variation from regular baked chicken: Cut your chicken into parts, place in a shallow pan and cover with crushed pineapple and sliced mushrooms and bake at 350 degrees for 1-1½ hours.

Chicken and ham go well together, as in the following dish: Take four large chicken breasts, skin and slice lengthways halfway through. Stuff with a thin slice of ham and one teaspoon blue cheese. Tie closed with nylon thread. Brush with melted margarine and enclose in foil. Bake in a moderate oven (350 degrees) for an hour. Remove the foil and roll each breast in wheat germ after taking off the thread. Serve topped with cranberries. Only about 210 calories per serving, plus all that good protein!

Chicken á la King seems to have gained a reputation for being the ideal way to handle leftover chicken, which may be true; but with a little imagination, it will taste more like its name—fit for a king. Here is the basic recipe:

Place one tablespoon margarine in a skillet and add 1 cup of finely chopped fresh onion. Cook over gentle heat for about 15 minutes; the margarine should not be so hot as to make the onion brown or crisp. You want the onions cooked, but still clear and clean looking. Now add the following ingredients: 4 cups chopped, cooked chicken (no skin!); 1 cup chicken bouillon; 2 teaspoons sea salt; ¼ teaspoon pepper; ¼ teaspoon thyme; ¼ teaspoon sweet basil; simmer gently for one minute. Now add the following ingredients, mixed in a blender: ½ cup skim milk; 2 hardboiled eggs; ¼ cup arrowroot or cornstarch. Pour in and cook gently until the mixture bubbles and thickens, about two minutes. Serve over rice or toast.

At your discretion, you may add: chopped parsley, chopped celery, a cup of sliced mushrooms, 4 tablespoons chopped green peppers, sliced pimiento or two tablespoons dry sherry for an extra special flavor treat! Let yourself go with any of the low-calorie vegetables and make your Chicken á la King something more than just a leftover dish. The above basic recipe should make about 8-10 servings of around 240 calories each.

Fish

We cannot stress too highly the value of whitefish for the dieter. Nothing is lower in fat and higher in protein—when properly prepared. Restaurants are notorious for soaking fish in batter, heavy in starch and absorbed fat, or drowning fish in a rich sauce overloaded with calories. But at less than 400 calories a pound, whitefish has no competition as a valuable food source that's ideal for the dieter, and the following recipes give you ample opportunity to prepare a wide variety of dishes that will tempt even the most lethargic fish-eater!

How about heavenly halibut for starters? The following recipe provides 4 servings at only 160 calories each: Take one pound of fresh halibut fillets, cut into convenient sized pieces and place in a shallow baking pan. Shake over fish: ½ teaspoon sea salt; ¼ teaspoon pepper, ¼ teaspoon paprika. Cover with a mixture of 1 chopped, peeled lemon and 10 chopped olives. Place a slice of tomato on each piece of fish and sprinkle with chopped parsley. Cover with aluminum foil and bake at 400 degrees for ten minutes; remove the foil and continue baking for another 20 minutes. May be served with a topping of yogurt sprinkled with wheat germ.

Italian-style white fish is great—tasting terribly rich, but in actuality having only 135 calories per serving. With 1½ pounds of fish, you should get around 6 servings. Use either flounder or perch. Cut the fish into small pieces and arrange in small clumps in a deep baking dish; we suggest you use lecithin to prevent sticking. Sprinkle with sea salt and pepper and douse with fresh lemon juice. Cover with aluminum foil and bake in a moderate oven (350 degrees) for fifteen minutes, by which time the fish should flake easily when tested with a fork. Pour off the liquid (water and lemon juice and fish nutrients) and place in a small saucepan. If necessary, add water to make about ¾ cup liquid. Bring to a boil and stir in ¼ cup skim milk and enough arrowroot or cornstarch to thicken (about 1 tablespoon) and remove from heat.

Now take 3-4 cups of cooked, chopped spinach, arrange around the clumps of fish in the baking dish, pour over the sauce and top with ¼ cup of grated Parmesan cheese. Pop into a hot oven (425 degrees) for about five minutes, or until the sauce bubbles. Remove at once and serve. If desired, you may substitute another green vegetable for the spinach, such as broccoli or green beans.

You can turn low-calorie fish into an extra-special dinner dish that will draw raves from guests and family alike. The following recipe serves 8 persons at just over 180 calories per serving: You will need 2 pounds of flounder fillets, spread out flat and trimmed into 8 pieces. Spread over each fillet the following mixture: ¾ cup chopped mushrooms; 3 tablespoons minced onion; 1 7½ ounce can of crabmeat, drained and chopped; ¼ cup wheat germ; 1 tablespoon chopped parsley; ½ teaspoon sea salt; ¼ teaspoon pepper. This mixture should be thoroughly mixed together in a bowl before spreading over each flounder fillet. After spreading evenly, roll up each flounder and place seam-side-down in a shallow baking dish. Any excess mixture can be placed around each fillet.

Now prepare a sauce with the following: 1½ cups skim milk; ¼ cup dry white wine; ½ teaspoon sea salt; 3 tablespoons arrowroot, cornstarch or whole wheat flour for thickening. Stir while the sauce thickens, bubbles and then add ½ cup shredded Swiss cheese. Continue stirring until the cheese melts. Pour over the flounder fillets, top lightly with paprika and bake in a hot oven (400 degrees) for 30 minutes, or until the flounder flakes easily when tested with a fork. Devastatingly delicious!

Whitefish need not be poached or steamed to keep down the calories. You can oven-fry any whitefish by rolling in a wheat germ mixture of ½ cup wheat germ to 2 tablespoons vegetable oil, plus sea salt and pepper to taste and a little paprika or chopped parsley for color. Place on a nonstick pan at 450 degrees for about 12 minutes, or until the fish flakes when tested. A serving of sole, flounder or perch cooked this way adds up to only 140 calories.

A final taste hint: To add a healthful crunch to whitefish, poached or baked, cover with a tablespoon of sprouts mixed with chopped parsley.

Vary Your Main Courses

Variety *is* the spice of life, particularly in a dinner menu, and going on a diet need not restrict your type of dish—only how you *cook* it, what you put *in* it, and how *much* you have of it!

Including natural food items in as many of your own recipes as possible will improve the protein and nutritional value of your menu, and watching the calorie level of each item will enable you to come out within whatever prescribed limits you have set for yourself. This may take a little more pre-planning than you usually give to your cooking, but once you have a daily menu laid out ahead of time, you can shop accordingly and cook accordingly. Although we recommend whitefish over beef for a dieter, because of the high protein and lower fat content, there is no reason to eliminate beef from your dinner, as long as you stick to low-calorie preparation as we have shown in the preceding examples.

Chapter Eight

Soups, Salads and Vegetables

We have stressed that preserving the natural
nutrients in food requires a little extra care in
menu planning and preparation: By cooking
ahead of time and freezing, you can eliminate a
lot of the work attached to mealtimes and also
reduce calories, as you will see in the following
directions for low-calorie soups. The right method
of vegetable cooking is also important in a natural food diet, helping to preserve the goodness,
vitamins and minerals that are vital to maintaining and restoring healthy tissue. Just as you are
required to put forth extra effort in counting
calories and carbohydrates in addition to selecting
your food items, so also must you pay attention
to cooking time of vegetables as well as meats.
Even organically-grown vegetables can be ruined
by improper handling, storage and cooking. All

aspects of menu planning must therefore be considered when you decide to give your family the benefits of natural foods.

Soups

Soup is a year-round dish, particularly popular for lunch—and highly recommended for dieters. Not only is a cup of soup warming and filling, but it helps provide nutrition and that satisfied feeling dieters often need psychologically.

For those who opt for the six-small-meals-a-day, soup can be used as a mid-afternoon or mid-evening snack; the plain soups, that is. The heartier soups that include meat and vegetables in addition to the liquid can be used as a main lunch or dinner course, depending on your taste and preference, and, of course, on your caloric limitations.

Here is a great recipe for a tasty soup that includes meat and vegetables, making it ideal for lunch: One cup of the liquid, plus ½ cup of meat, and ½ cup of vegetables totals less than 300 calories: You may choose between beef or chicken. For a beef soup, use 3 pounds of lean beef. For chicken, use two whole chickens.

Use a large Dutch oven or the traditional wide, deep stockpot. Place the meat in, together with the following ingredients: 1 tablespoon of sea salt; 1 tablespoon soy sauce; 3 quarts of water or, better yet, water you have used in cooking vegetables. We recommended earlier that you save all liquids from vegetable cooking, providing you with extra mineral and nutritional content for soups or stews.

Bring to a boil and simmer for four hours. Remove the meat (beef or chicken) and place the liquid in the refrigerator or freezer long enough for fat to rise to the surface and be skimmed off. While waiting, cut your meat into small chunks about one inch square, and, of course, remove any obvious pieces of fat.

Replace your cut-up meat in the cold liquid, together with three cups of chopped vegetables, such as carrots, green beans, onions, celery, tomatoes; don't forget at least half a cup of sprouts. Alfalfa sprouts are excellent, adding a freshness that really perks up the flavor. Avoid vegetables and other additions high in calories, such as dry beans, corn, peas, barley, lentils, rice, potatoes or noodles.

Bring to a boil again and simmer for a half hour or longer. When serving, place one cup of the liquid in a large bowl, then add ½ cup of meat and ½ cup of vegetables.

Soup made ahead of time can be frozen by pouring individual portions into small foil containers or paper cups (12 to 16 ounce size) and placing in the freezer. Defrost in a double boiler.

For extra protein content in a soup, add two or three tablespoons of brewer's yeast shortly before serving; it takes experimenting to determine the right quantity for your particular taste. With creamed soups, add half a cup of softened soy grits or powdered milk.

Potatoes are usually prohibited for dieters, but for those who enjoy a good creamy potato soup, here is a recipe that makes 8-10 servings at just 100 calories each. Take 2 pounds of fresh potatoes (preferably organically grown), peel and cut into quarters, and boil until tender, about 25-30 minutes. Drain and place to one side.

Melt 1 tablespoon margarine in a large saucepan and add three tablespoons of finely chopped onion. Cook over low flame until tender. Add 3 cups of chicken bouillon, 3 cups of skim milk, and 1 teaspoon sea salt. Leave over the flame until the mixture is hot, but not boiling.

Place the cooked potatoes in a blender, together with a cup of the hot bouillon mixture, and liquefy. This results in a smooth blend of the potatoes, with no lumpiness. Continue until all the potatoes have been blended with the liquid. Place the complete mixture over heat and bring to a boil and simmer gently for five minutes. Serve piping hot or, if you prefer, chill for a tasty cold summer dish. Finely chopped green onions or chives may be sprinkled over the soup before serving, if desired. For added protein, don't forget half a cup of soy grits or powdered skim milk, though we have found the potato soup by itself is quite rich-tasting.

A recipe for a delicious Italian-style soup, yielding about 5-6 cups of soup at only 100 calories per cup, follows: Take one pound of fresh tomatoes and drop in boiling water for a few minutes, then slide the skins off. Place tomatoes in a blender and liquefy; then pour into a soup pot and add the following ingredients: 2 cups of beef bouillon; 2 cups of chicken bouillon; 1 tablespoon finely chopped fresh onion; 1 teaspoon sea salt; ½ teaspoon pepper; 1 teaspoon Worcestershire sauce; ½ cup chopped fresh celery; ½ cup fresh sprouts, preferably wheat for sweetness. Bring to a boil and simmer for 30 minutes. Remove from heat, and add 1 cup of skim milk. Serve at once, complete with a topping of grated Romano cheese.

New Englanders will love this one: low calorie

140

clam chowder *plus* mushrooms! Take two teaspoons of margarine, place in a pot and melt until fairly hot. Add four ounces of mushroom stems and pieces and cook for two minutes over medium heat. Now add the following: one 7 ounce can of clams (including the liquid), 1 small minced onion; 1 stalk of celery, finely chopped or minced; ¼ teaspoon ground cloves; 2 tablespoons rye sprouts. Stir rapidly while cooking. Add a little water if necessary. Cook for five minutes, then add the following: 1½ cups skim milk; 1 cup water; 1 tablespoon arrowroot or cornstarch; 1 teaspoon sea salt; a pinch of pepper and 1 teaspoon Worcestershire sauce. Turn up the heat and allow to cook gently, but not boil, for about a minute. Only 130 calories per cup.

Californians love Mexican foods, which are usually high in calories—but there is one dish from south of the border which has all the spiciness you would want, but only 60 calories per cup: the famous ice cold soup called Gazpacho. This makes a delightful snack between meals, especially in summer.

Take six or seven medium sized tomatoes, skin in boiling water, then liquefy in a blender. Place in a pot and add the following ingredients: 1 onion, minced; 1 clove of garlic, minced; 1 green pepper, finely chopped; 1 large cucumber, finely chopped; 1 tablespoon wine vinegar; 2 teaspoons olive oil; 2 teaspoons sea salt; ¼ teaspoon pepper. Heat to simmering (not boiling) for about two minutes. Place in refrigerator for several hours, during which time the soup will thicken by itself. Serve ice cold in a cup or bowl, along with a fresh green salad.

Another refreshing summer soup, served cold, is

a cucumber frost, containing only 25 calories per cup and made as follows: Place in a blender 2 cups chopped cucumbers; 1 cup chilled chicken bouillon; ½ cup skim milk; 1 teaspoon sea salt; 1 teaspoon fresh lemon juice; 1 teaspoon Worcestershire sauce. Liquefy and serve over crushed ice, garnished with parsley or a slice of cucumber.

Many variations of low-calorie soups can be made in small or large quantities by using beef or chicken bouillon (only around 10 calories per cup) as a base, then adding fresh or left-over vegetables that have been liquefied in a blender.

Salads

Many dieters regard salads as mandatory calorie-cutters that do not always appeal to the appetite. Admittedly, those who have been plagued with a lettuce leaf and one slice of tomato may shudder at the word "salad", but salads can be tasty, tempting and a high point of any meal provided they are prepared with imagination. The following suggestions are guaranteed to make a mouth-watering addition to a dinner table, as well as being low in calories.

How about the traditional Caesar salad—but with only 50 calories per serving? For 10-11 servings, use one large romaine lettuce (about 1 pound). Break into small pieces in a large salad bowl. Take 2 eggs and place in boiling water for one minute. Remove and break over the lettuce and toss rapidly. Shake the following ingredients together: 4 tablespoons fresh lemon juice; ¼ teaspoon prepared mustard; 2 tablespoons grated Parmesan cheese; 1 teaspoon sea salt; ¼ teaspoon pepper; 1 teaspoon finely chopped anchovy fillets;

1 tablespoon alfalfa sprouts; blend and add to the lettuce and toss rapidly. Add one cup of croutons, toss and serve.

To make croutons, toast two slices of whole wheat bread, cut into ½ inch squares and stir into a skillet containing 1 tablespoon vegetable oil and ½ teaspoon garlic salt. Continue stirring until all the oil has been absorbed by the bread, which should be crisp. Allow to cool before adding to salad.

Another popular favorite, Waldorf salad, is a good low-calorie dish. The following recipe makes 4 half-cup servings of only 40 calories each. Toss together: 1 cup diced celery; 1 tablespoon seedless raisins; 1 cup diced fresh apple (do not peel) ; 2 tablespoons yogurt; ½ cup wheat germ (optional). Spoon the mixture onto a cluster of lettuce leaves.

Cole slaw is a perennial favorite. We have two recipes, the first tangy, the second sweet; both yield only 60 calories per serving.

Tangy cole slaw: 1 cabbage (2 pounds), finely shredded; ½ cup low-calorie mayonnaise; ¼ cup yogurt; ¼ cup buttermilk; 2 tablespoons natural sweetener, such as carob syrup; 1½ tablespoons cider vinegar; 1 teaspoon sea salt; ¼ teaspoon pepper. Blend together thoroughly and allow to chill in the refrigerator for at least 2 hours before serving, or preferably overnight for added deep flavor. Remember: Always stir cole slaw before serving, especially if it has been sitting for a while.

Sweet cole slaw: 1 cabbage (2 pounds), finely shredded; 1 cup grated or shredded carrot; 1 can (8 ounces) crushed pineapple, with juice; 8 ounces yogurt; 1 tablespoon cider vinegar; 1 teaspoon garlic salt; ¼ teaspoon sea salt; a dash of pepper. Blend thoroughly and refrigerate overnight, or for at least 2 hours before serving.

If you want an even lower-calorie cole slaw, try the next recipe: only 33 calories a serving. The following quantities make 4 servings: 2 cups cabbage, finely shredded; ¼ cup finely chopped celery; ½ cup yogurt; 1 teaspoon cider vinegar; 2 teaspoons natural sweetener; ½ teaspoon sea salt; a pinch of pepper. Combine and chill overnight, for at least two hours before serving.

If your calorie limit can stand it, potato salad makes a tempting addition to any luncheon menu. The following recipe makes about 12 cups of 100 calories each. Cook six medium-sized potatoes, peeled and diced, until tender, but not pulpy, about 15 minutes; drain and cool. Add six hard-boiled eggs, mashed together with 2 chopped onions and ½ cup finely chopped green pepper, plus 1 tablespoon sea salt and 2 tablespoons fresh lemon juice. Stir and then add the following dressing: 4 tablespoons low-calorie mayonnaise which has been blended (in a blender, set at medium) with 4 tablespoons diced pimientos. The dressing should come out an appealing pinky-orange color. Garnish with chopped parsley or watercress. Chill before serving.

For a change, you may add the pimientos at the same time as the eggs, and blend the peppers with the mayonnaise in the blender, giving the dressing a pale lime-green color that is very appealing. Remember, especially in dieting, food must *look* as good as it tastes!

Cucumber salad is good for summer, and only 45 calories a serving: Combine in a bowl 2 tablespoons fresh lemon juice; ½ teaspoon sea salt;

144

1 teaspoon natural sweetener; ½ cup yogurt or buttermilk. Peel and slice thin two medium-sized cucumbers and mix in with the dressing. Chill several hours before serving.

Gelatin is excellent from a nutritive standpoint and also enables the imaginative dieter to make molded salads that contain fruit and raw vegetables encased in an appealing shape. Rather than make one large mold, we suggest you buy four or six small molds to make individual servings. These will not only keep better in the refrigerator, but look more appealing when placed on the plate. Here is a tempting looking and tasting gelatin salad featuring ham and peaches, enough for 4-6 servings at only a little over 30 calories each: Dissolve 1 envelope unflavored gelatin in ½ cup of chicken bouillon over a low flame. Remove from heat and allow to cool. Blend in ½ cup of minced ham and 3 tablespoons mayonnaise. Chill until the mixture just begins to thicken. Add two stiffly beaten egg whites, stirring thoroughly. Cover the bottom of an eight-inch square shallow pan with slices of peaches (use individual molds if preferred) and spoon the mixture over the top. Place in refrigerator for 3-4 hours until set. Delicious served on a lettuce leaf with a garnish of chopped parsley or sprouts.

Many dieters turn a salad into a meal by the addition of their meat or fish allowance, finely chopped and mixed in with the green salad. Make sure you watch your measurements and check your calories and carhohydrates to stay within your limits!

Vegetables

We stress again: Prepare your own vegetable combinations, as well as sauces, and stay away from the pre-packaged frozen types that come complete with their own sauces. These commercially prepared sauces are not only high in preservatives and flavor-enhancers, but also are high in fats, starches and sugars—which means one package can often add up to more than 300 calories.

You can make the vegetable portion of your menu as exciting and imaginative as you want by varying your choice of vegetables, trying different ones *and* different combinations. There's no rule that says you can't dream up your own grab bag of color and flavor. Team up contrasting colors, like carrots with zucchini; broccoli with cauliflower and a smidgeon of tomato; peas with pumpkin; mushrooms, black olives and wild rice.

Vegetables are essential in everyone's daily diet, but only when properly prepared to preserve the inherent vitamins, minerals and general nutritive value; over-cooked vegetables are not only most unappetizing on the table, but cheat you out of the food value you need. So remember to steam vegetables as a general rule, or use a double boiler and let them cook in their own water. One commercial brand of frozen foods specializes in "five-minute" vegetables as though this were something revolutionary; this time limit applies to most vegetables, which should come out crispy and retaining their color. And, of course, organically-grown vegetables *do* possess more flavor, which you don't want to lose through careless cooking. Of course, most of us have to rely on the frozen food counter at the market, and while fresh frozen vegetables are acceptable, be sure to watch out for signs of deterioration.

Sometimes in the deliveries to a market, frozen items will thaw, and then be refrozen in the case. You can usually tell if this has happened by the pale, washed-out look of green vegetables, or a brownish cast to items like cauliflower. Always return such packages to the store for replacement. Freshness is essential to getting the most food value for your money, both in frozen and natural food items.

Consider various ways to vary your vegetables. For example, a grilled cheese sandwich can turn into a tasty surprise by using two slices of cheese, with a slice of fresh tomato between. As the sandwich browns on the griddle (or in your toaster oven) the cheese melts around the tomato. Does this give you further ideas of a similar nature? How about a tablespoon of sprouts between two slices of cheese? Or a teaspoon of cooked carrots and peas? Or even small pieces of left-over chicken or beef or ham? Just be sure to keep track of the amounts so you don't go over your calorie limit!

Varying the *way* you serve your vegetables can add interest to this essential part of your diet. For example, try baking tomatoes whole in their skins as a side dish. Just slice the tops off, and add a pinch of your favorite herbs, or half a teaspoon of Worcestershire sauce and a dab of margarine. Bake in a hot oven (400 degrees) until bubbly—5-10 minutes at the most.

Steamed celery sprinkled with paprika and bean sprouts makes a different and nutritious change. And don't forget many vegetables that you normally cook can also be used raw in salads: zuc-

147

chini, spinach, mushrooms, green beans or cauliflower can all add zest to a salad.

Similarly, for those who enjoy a sauce with a vegetable, you can achieve the same effect by cooking certain vegetables in bouillon to give extra flavor in place of a rich sauce. Broccoli is great cooked in beef bouillon. Green beans are delicious in chicken bouillon. If desired, you can thicken the bouillon with a teaspoon of arrowroot, which only adds 10 calories. Squash, cabbage, cauliflower and carrots also achieve a new piquancy by simmering in fruit juices, such as orange or lemon or apple. Again, arrowroot can be added for thickening into a tempting sauce.

Try to include high-protein, low-calorie items in cooking your vegetables: yogurt, for instance, can replace sour cream in cooking, and also cut the calories by 5 to 1! Here's a good recipe that adds a new dimension to cauliflower at less than 55 calories per serving. Take 4 cups of just-steamed cauliflower and place in a small casserole. Cover with 1½ cups of yogurt. Sprinkle with wheat germ, salt and parsley flakes. Bake at 425 degrees for 7-8 minutes, or until the wheat germ browns well. This recipe goes equally well with carrots, French-style green beans or broccoli.

A good Hollandaise-style low-calorie sauce can be made by placing in the top of a double boiler: 1 cup yogurt; 2 large egg yolks; 1 tablespoon fresh lemon juice; ½ teaspoon sea salt; a dash of pepper. Stir continuously until thick. This is especially good over brussels sprouts. Using two cups of this vegetable, you should get about six servings at around 70 calories each.

A delicious variation of yams is to mash them (after boiling) together with crushed pineapple, pop in a hot oven (around 400 degrees) for a half hour.

To vary your usual way of serving carrots, place the following ingredients in a blender: 3 cups cooked, chopped carrots; 3 egg yolks (save the whites) ; 2 tablespoons chopped chives; $\frac{1}{4}$ teaspoon nutmeg; $\frac{1}{2}$ teaspoon sea salt; $\frac{1}{4}$ teaspoon pepper. Blend thoroughly. Pour into a mixing bowl and add your three egg whites, after you have whipped them into firm peaks. Wipe a casserole dish with lecithin to prevent sticking and pour in the carrot blend. Put the casserole in a pan of water and bake in a moderate oven (350 degrees) for 45 minutes. This recipe gives about 8 servings at around 50 calories each. For a colorful garnish, sprinkle with finely chopped zucchini with bean sprouts.

Peas are usually considered too high in calories for most diets, but sharing the dish with other low-calorie items, they can add a flavorful and nutritious touch. The following recipe yields 8 servings at around 65 calories per serving: Sauté a pound of fresh, sliced mushrooms in a large skillet with one tablespoon of vegetable oil. Cook only 2 minutes, then add the following: 2 tablespoons fresh, chopped onion; 1 cup artichoke hearts; 1 cup green peas; 1 teaspoon garlic salt; $\frac{1}{2}$ teaspoon sea salt; 1 teaspoon chopped parsley; 1 cup chicken bouillon; a dash of pepper. Simmer gently for five minutes. Serve immediately.

With mixtures of vegetables, whether cooked on top of the stove or in the oven, remember never to overcook. In general, green vegetables should be slightly crisp when served. And for dieters, a general rule is to have at least *one* serving daily of raw vegetables in some form; the more, the better! Although careful cooking can still give you a nutritious helping of vegetables, remember the closer to nature you can get—meaning raw—the better.

Chapter Nine

A Week Of Easy Dieting

We have drawn up a daily diet for one entire week, Monday through Sunday, with a caloric limit of 1600 and the carbohydrates not exceeding 75 grams. We are including this to show you how you can still enjoy many mouth-watering recipes* and not go over your self-imposed limits. This illustrates how you can vary your diet from day to day. Do remember to get variety into your selection of foods, but, above all, watch the total number of calories and carbohydrates. It doesn't matter how you distribute them—maybe more for breakfast than for lunch, or more for dinner than for lunch. It's up to you, just as the three-meal-a-day routine often suits some people

*See index for individual recipes.

better than the six-a-day. But keep the carbohydrates under 75, no matter what; that's very important! If you get hunger pains, you can always nibble on some protein, such as cooked meat, whitefish, cheese, celery, radish, etc.—things that are low in carbohydrates. And keep track of those little snacks for calories and carbohydrates. If you don't, you're liable to wind up putting *on* weight instead of taking it off! The name of the game is counting calories and carbohydrates. Play by the rules and you'll wind up a winner. And by utilizing more natural foods in your daily menus, you'll increase the natural nutrients in your diet, a step in the right direction towards natural health and weight.

SUNDAY

	Calories	Carbo-hydrates
BREAKFAST		
3 slices crisp bacon	138	.6
1 square waffle	116	19.3
1 tablespoon dietetic maple syrup	22	5.1
Black coffee, tea or Sanka	0	.0
MIDMORNING SNACK		
½ cup cottage cheese topped with fresh peach	138	12.7
LUNCH		
6½ oz. light chunk tuna	294	0.0
on lettuce, tomato salad	45	7.0
1 slice whole wheat bread	55	11.9
Black coffee, tea or Sanka	0	.0
MIDAFTERNOON SNACK		
½ orange	36	9.5
DINNER		
1 slice roast beef	270	.0
One serving green beans	16	3.3
One serving zucchini	9	1.9
Black coffee, tea or Sanka	0	.0
EVENING SNACK		
4 oz. Swiss cheese	420	2.0
	1559	73.3

MONDAY

	Calories	Carbo-hydrates
BREAKFAST		
4 oz. fresh orange juice	56	12.9
2 egg/chicken bouillon omelet	190	3.0
3 slices bacon, broiled crisp	138	.6
1 slice whole wheat bread	55	11.9
Margarine for bread	25	.0
Black coffee, tea or Sanka	0	.0
MIDMORNING SNACK		
2 saltine crackers	24	4.0
Sanka	0	.0
LUNCH		
Jumbo hamburger (⅓ lb.) broiled	370	.0
Lettuce and tomato salad	45	7.0
1 slice whole wheat bread	55	11.9
Black coffee, tea or Sanka	0	.0
MIDAFTERNOON SNACK		
8—1" pieces celery stuffed with cream cheese	59	1.9
DINNER		
Cape Pot Roast—6 oz. serving	480	2.0
1 serving cooked carrots	25	5.8
1 tangerine	39	10.0
Black coffee, tea or Sanka	0	.0
EVENING SNACK		
¼ apple, sliced	17	4.0
	1578	75.0

TUESDAY

	Calories	Carbo-hydrates
BREAKFAST		
1 glass tomato juice (5½ oz.)	34	6.6
Baked cheese omelet	190	2.7
3 slices bacon, broiled crisp	138	.6
1 slice whole wheat bread	55	11.9
Margarine for bread	25	.0
Black coffee, tea or Sanka	0	.0
MIDMORNING SNACK		
3 oz. (½ cup) pineapple chunks	41	10.7
LUNCH		
Ham and egg sandwich	250	12.0
1 cup chopped lettuce (2 oz.)	8	1.7
1 teaspoon mayonnaise	25	.0
Black coffee, tea or Sanka	0	.0
MIDAFTERNOON SNACK		
2—1″ cubes American or cheddar cheese	138	.8
2 saltine crackers	24	4.0
DINNER		
Meat loaf—3 slices	300	9.2
1 serving (2.2 oz.) cauliflower, steamed	14	2.5
1 serving (2.4 oz.) carrots, diced, steamed	22	5.0
¼ apple, sliced, fresh	17	4.5
Black coffee, tea or Sanka	0	.0
EVENING SNACK		
1—8″ stalk of celery	7	1.6
	1288	73.8

WEDNESDAY

	Calories	Carbo-hydrates
BREAKFAST		
Buckwheat pancakes—4 pancakes	120	16.0
2 teaspoons dietetic maple syrup	44	10.2
2 poached eggs	160	.8
3 slices bacon, broiled crisp	138	.6
½ cup tomato juice	23	5.2
Black coffee, tea or Sanka	0	.0
MIDMORNING SNACK		
¼ cubed grapefruit	22	5.2
2 oz. Swiss cheese	210	1.0
LUNCH		
Chicken or turkey sandwich	260	12.8
½ cup grated raw carrot	23	5.2
Tea	0	.0
MIDAFTERNOON SNACK		
1 cup beef or chicken bouillon	12	2.2
2 saltine crackers	24	4.0
DINNER		
Beef stew (or curry)	220	5.6
4 spears steamed asparagus	12	2.2
1 serving mung bean sprouts	17	3.2
Black coffee, tea or Sanka	0	.0
EVENING SNACK		
4 oz. cooked shrimps	132	.8
	1417	75.0

THURSDAY

	Calories	Carbo-hydrates
BREAKFAST		
Sprout omelet	125	2.4
3 slices crisp bacon	138	.6
1 slice whole wheat bread	55	11.9
1 glass tomato juice (5½ oz.)	34	6.6
Black coffee, tea or Sanka	0	.0
MIDMORNING SNACK		
4 oz. fruit salad	57	13.3
2 pieces melba toast	18	3.0
LUNCH		
3 oz. beef liver with onion and apple	140	9.3
Lettuce and tomato salad	45	7.0
Black coffee, tea or Sanka	0	.0
MIDAFTERNOON SNACK		
4 oz. cooked shrimps	132	.8
DINNER		
Meat balls—large serving	340	9.2
Serving steamed broccoli	20	3.5
Serving steamed carrots	22	5.0
Coffee, tea or Sanka	0	.0
LATE EVENING SNACK		
4 oz. Swiss cheese	420	2.0
	1546	74.6

FRIDAY

	Calories	Carbo-hydrates
BREAKFAST		
German pancakes (1 serving)	200	13.6
3 slices bacon, broiled crisp	138	.6
¼ cubed fresh orange	20	4.0
Black coffee, tea or Sanka	0	.0
MIDMORNING SNACK		
½ chopped apple	35	9.1
2 oz. Swiss cheese	210	1.0
LUNCH		
8 oz. cooked shrimps	206	3.4
Lettuce and tomato salad	45	7.0
Black coffee, tea or Sanka	0	.0
MIDAFTERNOON SNACK		
½ cup yogurt	76	6.0
DINNER		
Beef and green vegetable loaf— large (double) serving	340	8.0
One serving cooked spinach (4 oz.)	27	4.3
One serving cooked crookneck squash (4 oz.)	15	3.2
Black coffee, tea or Sanka	0	.0
EVENING SNACK		
4 Vienna sausages	180	.0
4 saltines	48	8.0
	1540	68.2

SATURDAY

	Calories	Carbo-hydrates
BREAKFAST		
Curried eggs (2 eggs)	190	3.0
2 oz. cooked ham (lean)	72	.0
1 slice whole wheat bread	25	11.9
Margarine for bread	25	.0
Black coffee, tea or Sanka	0	.0
MIDMORNING SNACK		
½ grapefruit	44	11.7
LUNCH		
3 slices shepherd pie (meat only)	300	7.8
One serving French-style green beans	16	3.3
Black coffee, tea or Sanka	0	.0
MIDAFTERNOON SNACK		
4 Vienna sausages	180	.0
2 saltines	24	4.0
DINNER		
6 oz. baked flounder	340	.0
Lettuce, tomato and celery salad	53	8.0
1 slice whole wheat bread	55	11.9
Margarine for bread	25	.0
One tangerine	39	10.0
EVENING SNACK		
4 oz. boiled shrimps	132	.8
1 saltine	12	2.0
	1532	74.4

Chapter Ten

Count Those Calories and Carbohydrates!

While natural foods provide a sound basis for anyone's everyday diet, the person who wishes to lose weight *must* count calories and carbohydrates to shed those unwanted pounds, after which a sensible diet with the right amounts of natural foods will help you maintain a normal weight naturally.

There are many calorie guides on the market, but few list carbohydrates as well. We include the following listing which covers most items used in regular food preparation. Remember—check the count *before* cooking as well as *before* eating. Only you can determine what goes into your stomach—and what shows up on the scale later!

160

	Calories	Carbo-hydrates (GRAMS)
ACEROLA		
Fruit, with seeds (½ lb.)	52	12.6
Juice (½ cup)	28	5.8
ALMONDS		
Shelled (1 cup) 850		13.8
Salted (10 nuts)	83	2.7
ANCHOVIES (4 canned fillets)	28	less than .1
APPLE (1 medium)	70	20.0
APPLE BUTTER (1 tbsp.)	33	7.6
APPLE JUICE (1 cup, bottled or canned) 120		30.0
APPLESAUCE		
Canned, sweetened (1 cup) 230		60.0
Unsweetened or diet-pack (1 cup) ..100		26.0
APRICOTS		
Fresh (3)	55	13.7
Canned halves in heavy syrup (½ cup) 110		27.7
Canned diet-pack (½ cup)	56	14.9
Dried (10 halves) 140		40.0
APRICOT NECTAR (1 cup canned) ..140		36.0
ARTICHOKES		
Fresh, cooked (1 medium)	30	6.0
Frozen hearts, cooked (½ cup)	22	4.8
ASPARAGUS		
Fresh, cooked (6 spears)	20	3.0
Canned (6 spears)	20	3.3
Frozen, cut, cooked (½ cup)	18	3.2
Frozen spears, cooked (5 spears)	23	4.3
AVOCADO		
Fresh (½ medium) 370		13.0
Fresh, cut in cubes (½ cup)	97	6.7
BACON		
Broiled or fried crisp (2 slices) 100		.4
Canadian, lean, broiled (3 slices)	50	Trace

	Calories	Carbo-hydrates (GRAMS)
BAMBOO SHOOTS		
Canned (1 cup)	41	6.8
Raw, whole, untrimmed (½ lb.)	18	3.4
BANANA (One 6″ long)	85	21.1
BARLEY (pearl, uncooked, ¼ cup)	177	39.4
BEANS		
Baked with pork and molasses (1 cup)	302	52.0
Baked with pork and tomato sauce (1 cup)	295	48.4
Green, fresh cut, cooked (½ cup)	15	3.3
Canned, cut (½ cup)	14	4.1
Frozen, cut, cooked (½ cup)	18	4.6
Italian, frozen, cooked (½ cup)	23	4.1
Kidney, canned (1 cup)	230	42.0
Lima, baby, fresh, cooked (1 cup)	180	25.3
Mung, dry (½ cup)	357	63.3
Lima, dried, large, cooked (1 cup)	260	48.6
Fordhook, frozen, cooked (½ cup)	90	17.9
Wax, fresh, cooked (½ cup)	15	3.7
Wax, canned (½ cup)	15	3.2
Wax, frozen, cooked (½ cup)	22	5.0
BEAN SPROUTS		
Mung, boiled (½ cup)	17	3.2
Soy, boiled (4 oz.)	43	4.2
BEEF		
Brisket, fresh (1 slice— 7″ x 1½″ x ½″)	266	.0
Corned (1 slice—7″ x 1¼″ x ½″)	266	.0
Pot roast, blade (1 slice— 4″ x 3″ x ½″)	506	.0
Rib roast (1 slice—5″ x 3½″ x ¼″)	243	.0
Rump (1 slice—5″ x 5″ x ¼″)	235	.0
Sirloin (1 slice—5″ x 5″ x ¼″)	186	.0
Steak, cubed (12 oz. raw)	793	.0
Steak, club (6 oz. raw)	305	.0

	Calories	Carbo- hydrates (GRAMS)
BEEF—(Continued)		
Steak, flank (3 slices—5" x 1½" x ¼")	200	.0
Porterhouse (1 slice—4" x 3" x 1")	412	.0
Round (1 slice—6" x 4" x ½")	406	.0
Ground, raw (6 oz.)	271	.0
Ground sirloin (1 slice—4" x 3" x 1")	353	.0
Stew meat, chuck, boneless, raw (4 oz.)	421	.0
BEEF AND VEGETABLE STEW (1 cup, canned)	210	17.4
BEEF BROTH		
Canned, condensed, undiluted (1 can)	66	5.0
Cubes (1)	6	.5
Instant (1 envelope)	8	.5
BEEF (3 oz. canned corned beef)	185	.0
BEEF HASH (3 oz. canned, corned)	155	7.4
BEER (1 cup)	100	8.0
BEETS (1 cup fresh, cooked, diced)	50	12.2
BISCUITS (one 2½" baking powder)	129	14.0
BLACKBERRIES		
Fresh (½ cup)	43	9.4
Frozen, unsweetened (½ cup)	55	12.9
BLUEBERRIES		
Fresh (½ cup)	43	11.2
Frozen, unsweetened (½ cup)	45	11.2
Frozen, sweetened (½ cup)	129	30.2
BOLOGNA (1 slice)	87	.5
BRAN FLAKES (¾ cup)	95	22.9
BRANDY (1½ oz.)	75	Trace
BRAZIL NUTS (14 shelled)	100	1.9
BREAD		
Boston brown (1 slice)	100	21.9
Cracked wheat (1 slice)	60	12.0

	Calories	Carbo-hydrates (GRAMS)

BREAD—(Continued)
Bread items and other foods with calories and carbohydrates.

	Calories	Carbohydrates (grams)
BREAD—(Continued)		
French (1 slice)	108	15.0
Italian (1 slice)	108	18.0
Pumpernickel (1 slice)	65	12.4
Raisin, unfrosted (1 slice)	60	13.4
Rye (1 slice)	55	13.0
White, enriched (1 slice)	60	11.6
Whole wheat (1 slice)	55	12.3
BROCCOLI		
Fresh, spears, cooked (4)	40	8.6
Frozen, chopped, cooked (½ cup)	25	22.4
Frozen, spears, cooked (2-3)	26	3.6
BROWNIES (One 1½" x 1½" x ½")	120	17.0
BRUSSELS SPROUTS		
Fresh, cooked (1 cup)	56	9.9
Frozen, cooked (1 cup)	29	7.0
BUTTER (1 tbsp.)	100	less than .1
BUTTERMILK (1 cup, made from skim milk)	90	9.6
CABBAGE		
Raw, finely shredded (1 cup)	25	4.9
Cooked, finely shredded (1 cup)	35	6.2
Chinese, raw, chopped (1 cup)	15	2.2
CAKES		
Angel (1 slice—2")	110	24.1
Chocolate, with chocolate icing (1 slice—2")	445	67.0
Cupcakes, with chocolate icing (1 slice—2-3" diameter)	185	29.7
Plain, without icing (1 slice— 3" x 2" x 1½")	200	23.8
Poundcake (1 slice—3" x 2½" x 1")	140	14.1
Spongecake (1 slice—2")	120	28.6
CANDY		
Chocolate almonds (6)	102	10.8

	Calories	Carbohydrates (GRAMS)
CANDY—(Continued)		
Caramels (1)	42	8.4
Chocolate creams (1)	47	9.1
Chocolate fudge (1 piece— 1½" x 1½" x ½")	66	9.8
Chocolate mint (1—1½" diameter)	40	8.1
Marshmallows (1 large)	26	5.8
Peanut brittle (1 piece)	125	21.7
CANTALOUPE (½ medium)	60	14.0
CARROTS		
Raw, whole (one 5" x 1")	20	4.8
Raw, grated (1 cup)	45	10.6
Cooked, diced (1 cup)	45	10.0
CASABA MELON (4 oz.)	31	7.4
CASHEW NUTS (8, roasted)	164	8.3
CATSUP (1 tbsp.)	15	3.8
CAULIFLOWER		
Raw, flowerets (1 cup)	25	4.4
Cooked, flowerets (1 cup)	25	5.0
Frozen flowerets, cooked (½ cup)	15	3.0
CELERY		
Raw, diced (1 cup)	15	4.0
Raw, stalk (1)	5	1.6
Cooked, diced (½ cup)	12	2.4
CHARD (½ cup, boiled)	17	3.2
CHEESE		
Blue or Roquefort (1 oz.)	105	.6
Camembert (1 oz.)	86	.5
Cheddar or American (1 inch cube)	70	.4
Grated Cheddar or American (1 cup)	445	2.3
Cottage, skim milk, cream style (1 cup)	240	4.7
Cottage, dry (1 cup)	195	6.2
Cream (1 oz.)	105	.6
Parmesan, grated (1 tbsp.)	31	.2

	Calories	Carbo- hydrates (GRAMS)
Swiss, natural (1 oz.)	105	.5
CHERRIES		
Sour, red, canned (1 cup)	230	60.1
Sweet, fresh (1 cup)	80	20.4
Canned, sweetened (½ cup)	112	29.0
Canned, diet-pack (½ cup)	57	13.1
CHICKEN		
Broiled (½ broiler)	248	.0
Fried (½ breast)	201	1.1
Fried (1 drumstick)	101	.5
Roast (½ breast)	200	.0
Roast (1 drumstick)	101	.0
Roast (1 thigh)	147	.0
CHICKEN BROTH		
Canned (14 oz.)	74	.3
Cubes (1)	6	.4
Instant (1 envelope)	10	1.9
CHILI CON CARNE		
Canned, with beans (1 cup)	335	30.5
Canned, without beans (1 cup)	510	14.8
CHILI SAUCE (1 tbsp.)	17	3.8
CHOCOLATE		
Unsweetened (1 oz.)	145	8.2
Semi-sweet (1 oz.)	130	16.2
Sweet, cooking (1 oz.)	150	18.0
Bar, milk, plain (1 oz.)	150	18.9
Syrup, thin (1 tbsp.)	50	11.9
CLAMS		
Raw, meat only (4 large)	65	1.7
Canned, clams and liquid (4 large)	45	3.2
Juice (1 cup)	45	5.0
COCOA POWDER (1 tbsp.)	21	2.9
COCONUT		
Fresh (1 piece—2″ x 2″ x ½″)	161	4.2
Shredded (1 cup)	335	12.1
Dried, shredded, sweetened (1 cup)	340	30.0

	Calories	Carbo-hydrates (GRAMS)
COD		
Fresh poached (1 piece— 3″ x 3″ x 1″)	84	.0
Frozen, fillets, poached (4 oz.)	84	.0
COLA (1 cup)	95	20.0
COOKIES		
Chocolate wafer (one 2½″ diameter)	36	4.8
Creme sandwich, chocolate (1)	54	10.4
Fig bars (1 small)	55	13.8
Ginger snaps (one 3″ diameter)	52	8.6
Sugar wafer (one 2″ x ½″ x ¼″)	10	2.1
Vanilla wafer (1 average)	18	2.6
CORN FLAKES		
Plain (1 cup)	100	24.7
Pre-sweetened (¾ cup)	110	36.5
CORN (SWEET)		
Fresh, cooked (1 ear—5″)	70	16.2
Canned, cream style (½ cup)	92	22.5
Canned, whole kernel (½ cup)	70	17.0
Frozen, whole kernel, cooked (½ cup)	73	17.1
Frozen, on the cob, cooked (1 ear)	100	21.7
CORN MEAL (1 cup dry)	420	90.9
CORN OIL (1 tbsp.)	125	.0
CORN SYRUP (1 tbsp., light or dark)	60	15.8
CORNSTARCH (1 tbsp.)	30	7.0
COTTON SEED OIL (1 tbsp.)	125	.0
CRAB MEAT (3 oz.)	89	1.1
CRACKER MEAL (1 tbsp.)	45	7.1
CRACKERS		
Cheese (10—1″ sq.)	34	.3
Graham, plain (1—2¼″ sq.)	30	5.1
Chocolate graham (1—2″ sq.)	56	7.0
Oyster (20)	60	12.0
Rye wafers (2—3½″ x 1½″)	21	3.9
Saltines (1—2″ sq.)	14	2.2

	Calories	Carbo-hydrates (GRAMS)
CRACKERS—(Continued)		
Soda (1—2½″ sq.)	23	3.9
CRANBERRY JUICE COCKTAIL		
(1 cup, bottled)	160	39.4
CRANBERRY SAUCE (1 tbsp., sweetened, canned, jellied or whole berry)	26	6.1
CREAM		
Half-and-half (1 tbsp.)	20	.7
Whipping (1 tbsp.)	55	.5
Light (1 tbsp.)	30	.5
Sour, dairy (1 tbsp.)	29	.6
CRESS (1 lb. raw, whole, untrimmed)	103	17.7
CUCUMBER (one—7″ x 2″ raw, whole)	30	7.4
CUSTARD (1 cup, baked with whole milk)	285	29.2
DATES		
Dry, diced (1 cup)	490	126.8
Whole (4 oz.)	311	82.7
DOUGHNUTS (1 cake type)	125	16.4
DUCK (3 slices—3½″ x 2½″ x ¼″—roasted)	165	.0
EGG		
Whole (1)	80	.4
White (1)	15	.3
Yolk (1)	60	.1
ENDIVE		
Belgian (1 stalk)	10	1.1
Curly or chicory, broken (1 cup)	5	.8
Escarole (2 leaves)	5	1.4
FARINA (1 cup, cooked)	100	21.2
FENNEL LEAVES (one lb., raw, untrimmed)	118	21.5
FIGS		
Fresh (3 small)	90	22.4

168

	Calories	Carbo-hydrates (GRAMS)
FIGS—(Continued)		
Canned in syrup (½ cup)	115	30.3
Canned, diet-pack (½ cup)	68	14.1
Dried (2 medium)	100	29.0
FLOUNDER		
Fillet, fresh, poached (1 piece— 4″ x 2″ x 1″)	170	.0
Frozen, poached (4 oz.)	76	.0
FLOUR		
All-purpose, enriched, sifted (1 cup)	400	84.8
Cake or pastry, sifted (1 cup)	365	88.0
Self-rising, enriched (1 cup)	385	86.0
Whole wheat (1 cup)	400	80.4
FRANKFURTER (1)	120	.8
FRUITCAKE (1 piece—2″ x 2″ x ½″—dark)	115	17.9
FRUIT COCKTAIL		
Canned in syrup (1 cup)	195	50.4
Canned, diet-pack (½ cup)	60	32.0
GELATIN (1 tbsp., unflavored)	35	.0
GELATIN DESSERT		
Flavored, ready-to-eat (½ cup)	81	18.7
Low-calorie (½ cup)	9	Trace
GIN (2 oz.)	105	Trace
GINGERBREAD (1 piece— 2″ x 2″ x 2″)	175	28.6
GRAPEFRUIT		
Fresh (½ medium)	55	11.7
Fresh sections (1 cup)	75	20.2
Canned sections (1 cup)	175	45.6
Canned, diet-pack (1 cup)	70	18.2
GRAPEFRUIT JUICE		
Fresh (1 cup)	95	22.2
Canned, unsweetened (1 cup)	100	24.4
Canned, sweetened (1 cup)	130	32.0

	Calories	Carbo-hydrates (GRAMS)
GRAPEFRUIT JUICE—(Continued)		
Frozen concentrate, sweetened (6 oz. can)	350	84.8
Frozen, unsweetened concentrate (6 oz. can)	300	71.6
GRAPES (1 cup, fresh Concord, Delaware, Niagara, Catawaba, Scuppernong, Malagam Muscat, Thompson seedless, Emperor, Flame Tokay)	95	22.4
GRAPE JUICE (1 cup, bottled or canned)	165	42.0
HADDOCK		
Fresh, broiled (1 piece— 4" x 3" x ½")	100	.0
Frozen, broiled (4 oz.)	88	.0
HALIBUT		
Fresh, broiled (1 piece— 4" x 3" x ½")	217	.0
Frozen, broiled (4 oz.)	144	.0
HAM		
Baked (1 slice—5" x 3" x ½")	53	.0
Boiled, sliced (1 oz.)	35	.0
HERRING (2 oz. pickled)	127	.0
HOMINY GRITS (1 cup, cooked)	120	24.1
HONEY, STRAINED (1 tbsp.)	65	16.5
HONEYDEW MELON (⅛ medium)	31	7.2
ICE CREAM		
Commercial chocolate (⅔ cup)	200	19.8
Vanilla (⅔ cup)	193	15.8
ICE MILK (⅔ cup, chocolate)	144	18.8
JAMS, JELLIES, PRESERVES (1 tbsp.)	55	14.0
KALE		
Cooked (1 cup)	30	4.4
Raw, leaves only, untrimmed (1 lb.)	154	26.1

	Calories	Carbo- hydrates (GRAMS)
KIDNEY		
Cooked beef (3 oz.)	118	.8
Cooked lamb (3 oz.)	111	.9
Cooked pork (3 oz.)	130	1.0
LAMB CHOP		
Loin, raw (6 oz.)	223	.0
Rib, raw (5 oz.)	240	.0
Shoulder, raw (5 oz.)	252	.0
Shank, raw (10 oz.)	275	.0
LARD (1 tbsp.)	125	.0
LEEKS (4 oz. chopped, cooked)	59	12.7
LETTUCE (1 lb.)	47	8.4
LEMON (1 medium)	20	6.1
LEMONADE		
Concentrate, frozen, sweetened		
(6 oz. can)	430	104.8
Reconstituted (1 cup)	110	26.2
LEMON JUICE (1 tbsp., fresh)	5	1.2
LIMEADE CONCENTRATE		
Frozen, sweetened (6 oz. can)	410	107.9
Reconstituted (1 cup)	105	27.2
LIME JUICE (1 cup, fresh)	65	22.1
LIVER		
Cooked beef (4 oz.)	260	6.0
Cooked calf (4 oz.)	296	4.5
Cooked chicken (4 oz.)	146	3.3
Cooked lamb (4 oz.)	296	3.2
Cooked pork (4 oz.)	273	2.8
LIVERWURST (1 slice)	100	.7
LOBSTER		
Fresh, boiled (¾ lb. in the shell)	108	.3
Canned, meat only (½ cup)	80	.3
MACARONI (1 cup, cooked)	155	32.2
MACARONI AND CHEESE		
(1 cup, baked)	470	40.2

	Calories	Carbo-hydrates (GRAMS)
MALT (1 oz. dry)	104	21.9
MANDARIN ORANGES		
Canned, in syrup (⅓ cup)	55	17.6
Canned, diet-pack (⅓ cup)	29	6.2
MANGO (1 medium)	133	39.7
MARGARINE (1 tbsp.)	100	less than .1
MAYONNAISE (1 tbsp.)	100	.3
MELBA TOAST (1 slice)	17	3.0
MILK		
Whole (1 cup)	160	12.0
Skim (1 cup)	90	12.5
Condensed, sweetened (1 cup)	980	166.2
Dry, instant non-fat (1 cup)	330	47.6
Evaporated (1 cup)	345	24.4
Chocolate (1 cup)	205	27.5
MIXED VEGETABLES (½ cup frozen, cooked)	55	12.2
MOLASSES (1 tbsp.)	50	13.3
MUFFINS (one 2½" plain)	140	15.8
MUSHROOMS		
Fresh (6 large)	14	2.8
Canned, with liquid (1 cup)	40	4.1
Frozen, raw (14 cups)	10	1.9
MUSTARD (1 tbsp., prepared)	8	.5
NECTARINES (1 medium)	50	12.0
NOODLES (1 cup, egg, cooked)	200	37.3
OAT CEREAL (1 cup ready-to-eat)	100	19.0
OATMEAL (1 cup)	130	26.8
OKRA		
Fresh, cooked (8 pods)	25	5.3
Frozen, sliced, cooked (½ cup)	26	6.1
OLIVES		
Green, unpitted (4 medium)	15	.2
Ripe, unpitted (2 large)	15	.3
OLIVE OIL (1 tbsp.)	125	.0

	Calories	Carbo-hydrates (GRAMS)
ONION		
Green (6 small)	20	5.2
Raw, whole (1 medium)	40	8.7
ONION SOUP MIX (1 envelope)	150	23.2
ORANGE (1 medium)	70	19.0
ORANGE JUICE		
Fresh (1 cup)	110	25.8
Canned, unsweetened (1 cup)	120	27.8
Frozen concentrate, sweetened (6 oz. can)	330	80.9
Reconstituted (1 cup)	110	26.6
OYSTERS (13-19 raw, medium)	160	8.2
PANCAKES		
Plain, home-style (with egg and milk, 1-4″ diameter)	60	9.2
Buckwheat with egg and milk (1-4″ diameter)	55	6.4
PAPAYA (1 cup, fresh, cubed)	70	18.2
PARSLEY (1 tbsp. fresh, chopped)	1	.3
PARSNIPS (1 cup, cooked, diced)	100	28.8
PEACHES		
Fresh, whole (1 medium)	35	9.6
Fresh, sliced (1 cup)	65	16.4
Canned, in syrup (2 halves and 2 tbsp. syrup)	90	23.5
Canned, diet-pack (2 halves and 2 tbsp. syrup)	54	15.1
Dried, uncooked (1 cup)	420	120.2
Cooked, unsweetened (1 cup)	220	58.0
Frozen, sweetened (⅓ cup)	99	22.5
PEACH NECTAR (1 cup, canned)	120	31.0
PEANUTS		
Roasted, salted (20 medium)	100	2.6
Chopped (1 tbsp.)	55	1.7
Dry-roasted (¼ cup)	170	5.4
PEANUT BUTTER (1 tbsp.)	95	3.9

	Calories	Carbo- hydrates (GRAMS)
PEA PODS (4 oz. boiled, drained)	49	10.8
PEARS		
Fresh, whole (1 medium)	100	25.4
Canned, in syrup (2 halves and 2 tbsp. syrup)	58	27.0
Canned, diet-pack (2 halves and 2 tbsp. syrup)	62	16.8
PEAR NECTAR (1 cup, canned)	130	31.7
PEAS		
Green, fresh, cooked (1 cup)	115	19.8
Canned (1 cup)	146	29.8
Frozen, cooked (½ cup)	60	9.9
PECANS (12 halves)	100	1.9
PEPPERS		
Sweet, green, raw (1 medium)	15	2.9
Green, raw, diced (½ cup)	16	3.6
Red, raw (1 medium)	20	2.4
PERSIMMONS (1 medium)	75	20.1
PICKLES		
Dill (one 5″)	15	3.0
Sweet (one 3″)	30	5.8
PIES (⅛ of a 9″ pie shell)		
Apple	290	33.7
Blueberry	255	39.2
Cherry	299	38.2
Custard	233	39.2
Lemon meringue	264	40.1
Mince	298	36.8
Pecan	479	53.8
Pumpkin	230	33.6
PIMENTOS (1 medium canned)	10	2.2
PINE NUTS (pignolias ½ cup)	671	13.2
PINEAPPLE		
Fresh, diced (1 cup)	75	21.4
Canned, crushed, in syrup (2 slices)	195	50.8
Canned, sliced, in syrup (2 slices) ..	90	27.0

	Calories	Carbo-hydrates (GRAMS)
PINEAPPLE—(Continued)		
Canned, tidbits, diet-pack (½ cup) ..	57	15.6
Frozen, cubes (1 cup)	200	54.6
PINEAPPLE JUICE		
Canned (1 cup)	135	33.4
Frozen, reconstituted (1 cup)	125	31.9
PLUMS		
Fresh, whole (1 medium)	25	6.9
Canned, in syrup (3 plums and 2 tbsp. syrup)	100	25.9
Canned, diet-pack (3 plums and 2 tbsp. syrup)	75	19.7
PORK		
Chop, rib, raw (6 oz.)	250	.0
Chop, loin, raw (6 oz.)	283	.0
Roast, loin (1 chop—1" thick)	330	.0
Luncheon meat (2 oz.)	165	.6
POPCORN		
Popped with oil and salt (1 cup)	40	5.3
Plain (1 cup)	24	4.6
Sugar-coated (1 cup)	135	25.5
POTATOES		
Baked without skin (1 medium)	90	20.9
Boiled, peeled, cooked (1 medium) ..	105	23.3
Boiled, peeled, raw (1 medium)	80	17.7
French-fried (10 pieces)	155	22.0
French-fried, frozen, heated (10 pieces)	125	19.2
Mashed with milk only (½ cup)	70	12.7
POTATO CHIPS (10—2" diameter)	115	10.0
PRETZELS (10 small sticks)	10	2.0
PRUNES		
Cooked, unsweetened (17-18 medium)	295	77.9
Uncooked (4 medium)	70	4.8
PRUNE JUICE (1 cup)	200	48.0

	Calories	Carbo-hydrates (GRAMS)
PUMPKIN (1 cup canned)	75	19.2
RADISHES (4 small)	5	1.4
RAISINS (1 cup)	460	127.0
RASPBERRIES		
Red, fresh (1 cup)	70	19.6
Canned, in syrup (½ cup)	100	23.0
Frozen, sweetened (½ cup)	115	30.5
RHUBARB (1 cup cooked with sugar)	385	90.0
RICE		
White, cooked (1 cup)	185	33.8
Brown, cooked (⅔ cup)	100	25.5
Wild, cooked (½ cup)	73	23.8
RICE CEREAL (1 cup ready-to-eat)	115	24.9
RICE, PUFFED (1 cup)	55	13.4
ROLLS		
Frankfurter (1)	120	21.2
French (1—4″ x 2″ x 2″)	118	25.7
Hamburger (1—3½″ diameter)	123	21.2
Parker House (1—3″ x 2″ x 1½″)	114	18.9
RUTABAGAS (½ cup, cubed, cooked)	25	7.1
RYE WAFERS (3 rectangular)	63	12.1
SALAD DRESSING		
Blue cheese, low-calorie (1 tbsp.)	15	.7
Blue cheese, regular (1 tbsp.)	80	1.1
French, low-calorie (1 tbsp.)	9	Trace
French, regular (1 tbsp.)	65	2.8
Thousand Island, low-calorie (1 tbsp.)	33	2.3
Thousand Island, regular (1 tbsp.)	75	1.9
SALAD OIL (1 tbsp.)	125	.0
SALAMI (3 slices)	130	.3
SALMON		
Fresh, steak, broiled (1 piece— 6″ x 3″ x 1″)	430	.0
Canned (½ cup)	120	.0
SARDINES (4, canned in oil)	100	1.2

	Calories	Carbo-hydrates (GRAMS)
SAUERKRAUT (1 cup, canned)	32	6.2
SCALLOPS (6 medium, sea, fresh, raw muscle only)	105	3.7
SESAME SEEDS (1 oz.)	165	5.0
SHERBET (1 cup, orange, made with milk)	260	59.4
SHORTENING (1 tbsp., vegetable)	110	.0
SHREDDED WHEAT BISCUIT (1)	94	18.7
SHRIMPS		
Fresh, poached (7 medium)	100	1.7
Canned (5 oz.)	167	.8
SOLE		
Fillet, fresh, poached (1 piece)	177	.0
Frozen, poached (4 oz.)	88	.0
SOUPS (1 cup, canned condensed, prepared following label instructions)		
Cream of asparagus	51	10.1
Bean with bacon	130	19.4
Beef broth	22	2.2
Beef noodle	55	8.2
Black bean	80	13.9
Cream of celery	85	8.9
Cheese	142	9.7
Cream of chicken	85	7.9
Chicken gumbo	48	7.4
Chicken noodle	54	8.2
Chicken vegetable	60	8.6
Chicken with rice	44	5.8
Chili beef	133	20.8
Clam chowder	60	12.9
Consomme	25	2.4
Cream of green pea	110	22.5
Minestrone	85	10.5
Cream of mushroom	113	8.5
Onion	52	5.3

	Calories	Carbo- hydrates (GRAMS)

SOUPS—(Continued)

Pepper pot	83	8.6
Cream of potato	105	13.1
Split pea	130	20.6
Tomato	73	14.0
Tomato rice	82	12.8
Turkey noodle	65	7.5
Turkey vegetable	73	8.0
Vegetable	63	9.6
Vegetable beef	61	12.8
SOYBEAN CURD (4 oz.)	82	2.7
SOY SAUCE (1 tbsp.)	10	2.0
SOYBEAN OIL (1 tbsp.)	125	.0
SPAGHETTI (1 cup, cooked)	155	32.2

SPINACH

Fresh, cooked (1 cup)	40	5.6
Canned (1 cup)	45	7.1
Frozen, chopped or leaf (1 cup)	24	4.3

SQUASH (yellow, zucchini,
crookneck, patty pan)

Sliced, cooked (1 cup)	30	4.8
Frozen, cooked (½ cup)	20	3.8

STRAWBERRIES

Fresh (1 cup)	55	12.1
Frozen, whole, sweetened (⅔ cup)	131	34.9
Whole, unsweetened, frozen (1 cup)	55	12.1
Sliced, sweetened, frozen (½ cup)	140	39.1
SUCCOTASH (½ cup, frozen, cooked)	87	19.7

SUGAR

Granulated white (1 tbsp.)	45	11.9
Brown (1 tbsp.)	51	12.5
Lump (1)	25	6.0
Confectioner's powdered (1 tbsp.)	23	5.9

SWEET POTATOES

Baked without skin (1 medium)	155	35.8

	Calories	Carbo-hydrates (GRAMS)
SWEET POTATOES—(Continued)		
Peeled, boiled (1 medium) 170		38.7
Canned, without syrup (1 cup) 235		45.0
SYRUP		
Corn, light or dark (1 tbsp.) 60		15.0
Maple (1 tbsp.) 61		13.0
Maple blended, low calorie (1 tbsp.) 21		5.5
Maple blended, regular, pancake, sorghum (1 tbsp.) 54		15.0
TANGERINE (1 large) 40		10.0
TANGERINE JUICE (1 cup, canned, unsweetened) 105		25.2
TAPIOCA (1 tbsp., quick-cooking, uncooked) 35		8.6
TOMATOES		
Fresh (1 medium) 35		7.0
Canned (1 cup) 50		10.2
TOMATO JUICE (1 cup, canned) 45		10.4
TUNA		
Canned in oil, drained (½ cup) 170		.0
Canned in water (½ cup) 109		.0
TURNIPS (1 cup, white, cooked) 35		7.6
TURKEY (1 slice—4" x 2½" x ¼"— roasted breast) 134		.0
VEAL		
Chop, loin, raw (8 oz.) 251		.0
Chop, rib, raw (6 oz.) 240		.0
Leg, roasted (1 slice—5" x 4" x ¼") 159		.0
VINEGAR (1 tbsp.) 1		.8
WALNUTS (1 tbsp., English, chopped) 50		1.2
WATER CHESTNUTS (4 oz. peeled) .. 90		21.5
WATERMELON (1 wedge— 4" x 4" x 8"—fresh) 115		27.3

	Calories	Carbo-hydrates (GRAMS)
WHEAT CEREAL		
Ready-to-eat flakes (1 cup)	248	56.4
Puffed (1 cup)	44	9.4
Puffed, pre-sweetened (1 cup)	45	10.6
WHEAT GERM (1 oz.)	106	12.6
YAMS (4 oz., raw, peeled)	115	26.3
YEAST, BREWER'S (1 oz., dry)	80	10.9
YOGURT		
Skim milk (1 cup)	120	12.6
Whole milk (1 cup)	152	12.0
ZWIEBACK (1 slice)	31	5.4

Remember: Stick to your guns and your diet—count those calories and carbohydrates, and when you find your courage failing, just step on the bathroom scale. Watching your weight come down is the greatest morale booster of all!

Be of good cheer and you'll soon be of good weight—the right, healthy weight you should be. And learn to stay that way by eating only the right amounts of the right *natural* foods.

Index

INDEX

INDEX

INDEX

INDEX

INDEX

(Tocopherol)
importance in diet,
35
sources of, 35
Vitamin F,
35
importance in diet,
sources of, 35
Vitamin H,
See Biotin
Vitamin K,
importance in diet,
35
sources of, 35
Vitamin M,
see Folic acid
Vitamin P
(Bioflavanoids)
importance in diet,
35
sources of, 135
Vitamins,
importance in diet,
21, 27, 28, 39
preservation of, 60,
61

—W—

Weight control,
with natural foods,
43, 44, 53
physical and
psychological
factors of, 9, 74,
75
Wheat germ, 51

—Z—

Zinc,
importance in diet,
38